Frontiers in Anti-Cancer Drug Discovery

(*Volume 11*)

Edited by

Atta-ur-Rahman, *FRS*

Honorary Life Fellow,
Kings College,
University of Cambridge,
Cambridge,
UK

&

M. Iqbal Choudhary

H.E.J. Research Institute of Chemistry,
International Center for Chemical and Biological Sciences,
University of Karachi,
Karachi,
Pakistan

Frontiers in Anti-Cancer Drug Discovery

Volume # 11

Editors: Atta-ur-Rahman and M. Iqbal Choudhary

ISSN (Online): 1879-6656

ISSN (Print): 2451-8395

ISBN (Online): 978-981-14-2213-3

ISBN (Print): 978-981-14-2212-6

ISBN (Paperback): 978-981-14-7009-7

need for a court order if at any point you breach any terms of this License Agreement. In no event will any delay or failure by Bentham Science Publishers in enforcing your compliance with this License Agreement constitute a waiver of any of its rights.

3. You acknowledge that you have read this License Agreement, and agree to be bound by its terms and conditions. To the extent that any other terms and conditions presented on any website of Bentham Science Publishers conflict with, or are inconsistent with, the terms and conditions set out in this License Agreement, you acknowledge that the terms and conditions set out in this License Agreement shall prevail.

Bentham Science Publishers Pte. Ltd.
80 Robinson Road #02-00
Singapore 068898
Singapore
Email: subscriptions@benthamscience.net

BENTHAM
SCIENCE

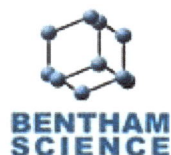

CONTENTS

PREFACE i

LIST OF CONTRIBUTORS ii

CHAPTER 1 PI3K/AKT/MTOR PATHWAY IN ACUTE LYMPHOBLASTIC LEUKEMIA
TARGETED THERAPIES 1
Carolina Simioni, Giorgio Zauli, Daniela Milani and Luca M. Neri
   INTRODUCTION 1
      Acute Lymphoblastic Leukemia 3
      PI3K/Akt/mTOR Signaling 5
      Aberrant PI3K/Akt/mTOR Expression in ALL 7
         PI3K Inhibition in ALL 8
         Akt Inhibition 10
         Classes of mTOR Inhibitors: Roles of Rapamycin, Rapalogs, Dual PI3K/mTOR
         Inhibitors and TORKIs 12
      Clinical Trials 19
         PI3K Inhibition 19
         Akt Inhibition 20
         mTOR Inhibition 20
   CONCLUDING REMARKS 21
   LIST OF ABBREVIATIONS 22
   CONSENT FOR PUBLICATION 23
   CONFLICT OF INTEREST 23
   ACKNOWLEDGEMENTS 23
   REFERENCES 23

CHAPTER 2 POLYMERIC NANOMEDICINES IN TREATMENT OF BREAST CANCER:
REVIEW OF CONTEMPORARY RESEARCH 36
*Farooq Ali Khan, Md. Rizwanullah, Ahmad Perwez, Mohammad Zaki Ahmad and
Javed Ahmad*
   INTRODUCTION 37
   CHALLENGES IN TREATMENT OF BREAST CANCER 37
   POTENTIAL OF POLYMERIC NANOMEDICINES IN TREATMENT OF BREAST
   CANCER 39
   TARGETING IN TREATMENT OF BREAST CANCER 41
      Passive Targeting 41
      Active Targeting 42
   DIFFERENT POLYMERIC NANOMEDICINES IN TREATMENT OF BREAST
   CANCER 43
      Polymeric Nanoparticles 43
      Polymeric Micelles 47
      Polymer-lipid Hybrid Nanoparticles 52
      Dendrimers 54
   POLYMERIC NANOMEDICINE FOR GENE THERAPY IN BREAST CANCER 58
   CONCLUDING REMARKS 60
   LIST OF ABBREVIATIONS 60
   CONSENT FOR PUBLICATION 61
   CONFLICT OF INTEREST 61
   ACKNOWLEDGEMENTS 61
   REFERENCES 61

CHAPTER 3 TREATMENT OF LUNG CANCER IN THE NEW ERA 67
Girisha Maheshwari, Bhanu Pratap Chauhan, Shweta Dang and *Reema Gabrani*
    INTRODUCTION 67
    SMALL MOLECULE-BASED INHIBITORS 68
        First Generation Inhibitors 70
        Second Generation Inhibitors 71
        Third Generation Inhibitors 71
    MONOCLONAL ANTIBODIES 72
    NOVEL APPROACHES 74
        Epigenetic Therapies 74
        MicroRNA 75
        Tumor Supressor MicroRNAs in Lung Cancer 75
        Oncogenic MicroRNA in Lung Cancer 75
    NANOPARTICLE FORMULATIONS 76
    PERSONALIZED MEDICINE 77
    CONCLUSION 77
    CONSENT FOR PUBLICATION 78
    CONFLICT OF INTEREST 78
    ACKNOWLEDGEMENTS 78
    REFERENCES 78

CHAPTER 4 ORAL ADMINISTRATION OF CANCER CHEMOTHERAPEUTICS
EXPLOITING SELF-NANOEMULSIFYING DRUG DELIVERY SYSTEM: RECENT
PROGRESS AND APPLICATION 83
*Javed Ahmad, Farooq Ali Khan, Mohammad Zaki Ahmad, Showkat Rasool Mir, Noor
Alam* and *Saima Amin*
    INTRODUCTION 84
    ANTICANCER ORAL THERAPY 85
    BIOPHARMACEUTICAL BARRIERS IN ORAL CHEMOTHERAPY 86
    SELF-NANOEMULSIFYING DRUG DELIVERY SYSTEM FOR ANTICANCER ORAL
    THERAPY 88
        Contemporary Research and Application 90
        Recent Progress and Advancement 93
            Solidification Technique Transforming SNEDDS into Solid Dosage Forms 94
            Challenges with Solidification Techniques 95
            Strategies to Overcome the Challenges Associated with Solidification Techniques 95
    CONCLUDING REMARKS 96
    CONSENT FOR PUBLICATION 96
    CONFLICT OF INTEREST 96
    ACKNOWLEDGEMENTS 96
    LIST OF ABBREVIATIONS 96
    REFERENCES 97

CHAPTER 5 TARGETING APPROACHES FOR THE DIAGNOSIS AND TREATMENT OF
CANCER 105
*Shivani Saraf, Ankita Tiwari, Amit Verma, Pritish K. Panda, Sarjana Raikwar, Ankit
Jain, Rupal Dubey* and *Sanjay K. Jain*
    INTRODUCTION 105
    DIAGNOSIS TECHNOLOGY 107
    RECENT APPROACHES FOR THE TREATMENT OF CANCER 111
        Targeted Drug Delivery Carriers 111

   Liposomes 111
   Nanoparticles 113
   Nanoemulsion 114
   Hydrogel 115
   Gene Therapy 116
   Aptamer Based System 117
   Antibody Based System 118
  Stimuli Sensitive Drug Delivery Systems 120
   pH Sensitive Drug Delivery Systems 121
   Temperature Sensitive Drug Delivery Systems 122
   Magnetic Sensitive Drug Delivery Systems 122
   Redox Sensitive Drug Delivery Systems 123
   Photosensitive Drug Delivery Systems 123
  Herbal Drug Approaches 124
CONCLUSION 127
CONSENT FOR PUBLICATION 127
CONFLICT OF INTEREST 128
ACKNOWLEDGEMENTS 128
REFERENCES 128

SUBJECT INDEX 139

PREFACE

Despite tremendous development in our understanding of different types of cancer at biochemical and genetic levels, prevention, diagnosis, and treatment is still far from perfect. Based on the histopathological heterogeneity and remarkable genetic complexities of cancer, research on this disease has emerged as a truly interdisciplinary science. From biomarker identification for diagnosis and diseases progression monitoring to personalized treatment, the research is spread over a wide range of fields and disciplines. This book series *"Frontiers in Anti-Cancer Drug Discovery"* is, therefore, aimed to provide comprehensively written review articles on carefully selected topics in this important field. Volume 11 of the book series contains five (5) chapters covering target identification to new classes of anticancer therapies, each contributed by eminent experts.

The review contributed by Neri *et al.* focusses on the importance of targeting phosphoinositide 3 kinases (P13Ks), their downstream mediator Akt and the mammalian target of rapamycin (mTOR) as targets for drug discovery against the acute lymphoblastic leukemia (ALL). They have included examples of small molecular inhibitors of P13Ks/Akt/mTOR as targeted drug candidates. Javed *et al.* have reviewed recent researches on polymeric nanomedicine for the treatment of breast cancers. The results of preclinical studies on polymeric nanomedicines in terms of target specificity, improved bioavailability and safety *via* their passive and active modes of action arepresented. Lung cancers (non-small cell lung cancer and small cell lung cancer) are among the most aggressive cancer types with high mortality. Gabrani *et al.* review recent developments in the treatment of lung cancers, including EGFR tyrosine kinase inhibitors (TKIs), inhibitors of imbalance microRNA, and immunotherapy. Saima *et al.* have contributed a comprehensive chapter on the recent advancements in the applications of self-nonemulsifying drug delivery system (SNEDDS) for cancer chemotherapeutics. SNEDDSs offer improved bioavailability and greater tolerability as oral anticancer drug delivery vehicles. Last but not the least, Jain *et al.* focus on exciting advances in novel targeting approaches for the prevention, diagnosis and treatment of cancers. This includes theranostics based systems for diagnosis coupled cancer therapies.

The above review articles by prominent researchers in the field of cancer research directed towards anticancer drug discovery should be of great interest to research scholars. We are grateful to all the authors for their excellent and scholarly contributions to the 11th volume of this internationally acclaimed ebook series. The Editorial team of Bentham Science Publishers deserves appreciation for the efficient processing and timely management of this publication. The coordination and liaison by Ms. Fariya Zulfiqar (Manager Publications), under the leadership of Mr. Mahmood Alam (Director Publications) is gratefully acknowledged. We also hope that like the previous volumes of this book series, the current compilation will also receive wide readership, and appreciation.

Prof. Dr. Atta-ur-Rahman, *FRS*
Honorary Life Fellow
Kings College
University of Cambridge
Cambridge
UK

Prof. Dr. M. Iqbal Choudhary
H.E.J. Research Institute of Chemistry
International Center for
Chemical and Biological Sciences
University of Karachi
Karachi
Pakistan

List of Contributors

Ahmad Perwez Genome Biology Lab, Department of Biosciences, Jamia Millia Islamia, New Delhi, India

Amit Verma Pharmaceutics Research Projects Laboratory, Department of Pharmaceutical Sciences, Dr. Hari Singh Gour Vishwavidyalaya, Sagar (M.P.) 470 003, India

Ankita Tiwari Pharmaceutics Research Projects Laboratory, Department of Pharmaceutical Sciences, Dr. Hari Singh Gour Vishwavidyalaya, Sagar (M.P.) 470 003, India

Ankit Jain Institute of Pharmaceutical Research, GLA University, NH-2, Mathura-Delhi Road, Mathura (U.P.) 281 406, India

Bhanu Pratap Chauhan Jaypee Institute of Information Technology, A-10, Sector 62, Noida, Uttar Pradesh, India

Carolina Simioni Department of Medical Sciences, University of Ferrara, Ferrara, Italy

Daniela Milani Department of Morphology, Surgery and Experimental Medicine, University of Ferrara, Ferrara, Italy

Farooq Ali Khan Sri Indu Institute of Pharmacy, Hyderabad, India

Giorgio Zauli Department of Morphology, Surgery and Experimental Medicine, University of Ferrara, Ferrara, Italy
LTTA Center- Flow Cytometry and Cell Sorting service, University of Ferrara, Ferrara, Italy

Girisha Maheshwari Jaypee Institute of Information Technology, A-10, Sector 62, Noida, Uttar Pradesh, India

Javed Ahmad Department of Pharmaceutics, College of Pharmacy, Najran University, Najran, Kingdom of Saudi Arabia (KSA)

Luca M. Neri Department of Morphology, Surgery and Experimental Medicine, University of Ferrara, Ferrara, Italy
LTTA - Electron Microscopy Center, University of Ferrara, Ferrara, Italy

Md. Rizwanullah Department of Pharmaceutics, School of Pharmaceutical Education and Research, Jamia Hamdard, New Delhi, India

Mohammad Zaki Ahmad Department of Pharmaceutics, College of Pharmacy, Najran University, Najran, Kingdom of Saudi Arabia (KSA)

Noor Alam Post-Graduate Department of Botany, Purnea University, Bihar, India

Pritish K. Panda Pharmaceutics Research Projects Laboratory, Department of Pharmaceutical Sciences, Dr. Hari Singh Gour Vishwavidyalaya, Sagar (M.P.) 470 003, India

Reema Gabrani Jaypee Institute of Information Technology, A-10, Sector 62, Noida, Uttar Pradesh, India

Rupal Dubey School of Pharmacy and Research, People's University, Bhopal (M.P.)462037, India

Saima Amin Department of Pharmaceutics, School of Pharmaceutical Education and Research, Jamia Hamdard, New Delhi, India

Sanjay K. Jain Pharmaceutics Research Projects Laboratory, Department of Pharmaceutical Sciences, Dr. Hari Singh Gour Vishwavidyalaya, Sagar (M.P.) 470 003, India

Sarjana Raikwar   Pharmaceutics Research Projects Laboratory, Department of Pharmaceutical Sciences, Dr. Hari Singh Gour Vishwavidyalaya, Sagar (M.P.) 470 003, India

Showkat Rasool Mir   Phytopharmaceutical Research Laboratory, School of Pharmaceutical Education and Research, Jamia Hamdard, New Delhi, India

Shweta Dang   Jaypee Institute of Information Technology, A-10, Sector 62, Noida, Uttar Pradesh, India

Shivani Saraf   Pharmaceutics Research Projects Laboratory, Department of Pharmaceutical Sciences, Dr. Hari Singh Gour Vishwavidyalaya, Sagar (M.P.) 470 003, India

CHAPTER 1

PI3K/Akt/mTOR Pathway in Acute Lymphoblastic Leukemia Targeted Therapies

Carolina Simioni[1], Giorgio Zauli[2,3], Daniela Milani[2] and Luca M. Neri[2,4,*]

[1] *Department of Medical Sciences, University of Ferrara, Ferrara, Italy*

[2] *Department of Morphology, Surgery and Experimental Medicine, University of Ferrara, Ferrara, Italy*

[3] *LTTA Center- Flow Cytometry and Cell Sorting service, University of Ferrara, Ferrara, Italy*

[4] *LTTA - Electron Microscopy Center, University of Ferrara, Ferrara, Italy*

Abstract: Acute Lymphoblastic leukemia (ALL) comprises a subset of different hematologic neoplasms characterized by impaired proliferation of immature lymphoid cells in bone marrow and peripheral blood. Pediatric patients have experienced treatment success with 5- year overall survival rates approaching 90%, whereas ALL adult patients are associated with poorer survival. Therefore, the development of new targeted therapeutic protocols constitutes a primary need. Phosphoinositide 3-kinases (PI3Ks) and their downstream mediators Akt and mammalian target of rapamycin (mTOR) represent the main components of the PI3K/Akt/mTOR signaling network. It is a key regulatory signaling cascade which drives proliferation, survival and drug-resistance of cancer cells, and it is frequently up-regulated in the different T- and B-ALL subtypes. Serious and irreversible late effects from conventional therapy are a growing issue for leukemia survivors, both for adult and pediatric patients. Therefore, the need to develop targeted and personalized therapy protocols for the treatment of leukemias is mandatory. Recent diagnostic tools allow to design therapeutic protocols with increased target specificity towards PI3K/Akt/mTOR axis that represents a critical target for cancer therapy. This chapter will focus on how this pathway could constitute a paradigm for the development of therapeutic strategies and how effective the recent pharmacological Small Molecule Inhibitors (SMIs) can suppress leukemic cell growth.

Keywords: Acute Lymphoblastic Leukemia, Apoptosis, Autophagy, Cytotoxicity, PI3K/Akt/mTOR, Proliferation, Signal transduction, Small Molecule Inhibitors (SMIs), Survival, Targeted Therapies, Tyrosine Kinase Inhibitors (TKIs).

INTRODUCTION

Neoplastic diseases such as solid tumors and leukemia hematological disorders

---

* **Corresponding author Luca M. Neri:** Department of Morphology, Surgery and Experimental Medicine, University of Ferrara, Ferrara, Italy; Tel; +39-0532-455940; E-mail: luca.neri@unife.it

Atta-ur-Rahman and M. Iqbal Choudhary (Eds.)

contribute significantly to morbidity and mortality of the population worldwide [1 - 4]. Whereas, some cancers show declining incidences in part due to effective prevention programs, others such as ALL are increasing in incidence. This is in part due to the fact that as life expectancy is increasing, in parallel some ALL incidence increases as well.

Development of new targeted treatment strategies aiming to increase cure rates and to decrease side effects is essential to take care of this patient population. Fundamental bases for such developments are a complex knowledge on oncogenesis, and more specifically on leukemogenesis [5, 6]. Aberrantly activated signaling pathways have been identified in different cancer models leading to the development of specific drugs, targeted therapies and ameliorated cure rates.

An example of aberrantly activated signaling pathways or receptors that could contribute to the oncogenesis mechanism is, in colon cancer cells, the Epidermal Growth Factor Receptor (EGFR). This receptor is responsible for the activation of RAS/RAF/MAPK pathway [7]. Subsequently, EGFR inhibitors and anti-EGF antibodies were developed, improving treatment outcomes. Similarly, in renal carcinoma, abnormal activation of receptor tyrosine kinases has been identified, leading to an abnormal activation of the VEGF/RAF/RAS pathway [8]. Other multikinase inhibitors, such as Regorafenib for colon cancer or Cabozantinib for renal carcinoma and hepatocellular carcinoma, have been developed with the aim to increase survival and quality of life [9 - 11].

It has been reported that in ALL, and especially in the T-ALL subtype, the EGFR pathway inhibition enhanced anticancer drugs induced cell death [12]. But another signaling pathway that displays constitutive activation in ALL, leading to uncontrolled production of malignant cells and driving chemotherapy resistance is the PI3K/Akt/mTOR signaling network. PI3K/Akt/mTOR is one of the most frequently aberrant activated pathway, and the inactivation of the tumor suppressor gene Phosphatase and tensin homolog (PTEN) represents one of the causes of this network stimulation [13 - 16], thereby giving the cancer cell a survival advantage. Indeed, literature data indicate that genetic alterations in components of PI3K/Akt/mTOR network have a close relationship with the development of ALL, thereby contributing to leukemogenesis, and these evidences highlighted the importance of developing new targeted therapies against this signaling network, with the aim to better predict favorable outcomes in acute leukemia patients. In chronic myeloid leukemia (CML), activation of this pathway is correlated to BCR-ABL tyrosine kinase, found also in 25% of adult ALL and less in ALL childhood. Treatment of ALL adults is more difficult than in pediatric patients due to the higher frequency of this chromosome rearrangement, including also the development of a recently characterized subtype, Philadelphia (Ph)-like ALL, with high expression of signaling tyrosine kinases, resulting in stimulation of Abl and the Janus kinase (JAK) signal transducer of activation (STAT) pathway (Jak/Stat) pathways [17]. As PI3K signaling is considered to be one of the decisive pathways for the transformation potential of BCR-ABL, and that it may play a role in causing one of the tyrosine kinase inhibitor (TKI) resistance, that is imatinib, the pharmacological combination of more than one targeted cascade inhibitor is necessary, as well as the association of drugs targeting the same pathway at multiple levels. Pediatric patients have better prognosis because of minimal residual disease (MRD) monitoring and the intensification of more targeted treatments that, in association also with recent PI3K/Akt/mTOR inhibitors, could overcome glucocorticoid (GC) treatment resistance, frequently observed in ALL pediatric patients.

The importance of targeting this signaling network will be discussed in this chapter, together with a detailed profile of the most recent PI3K/Akt/mTOR inhibitors, also known as SMIs, tested in preclinical and recent clinical studies for the treatment of ALL.

Acute Lymphoblastic Leukemia

ALL is a malignant hematological disorder characterized by aberrant expansion and diffusion in blood and bone marrow of lymphoid progenitor cells. ALL is the most frequent cancer identified in children [18].

Based on morphology and cytogenetic profiles, two different types of ALL have been identified: B-acute lymphoblastic (B-ALL) and T-acute lymphoblastic (T-ALL).

The uncontrolled growth of B-cell precursors represents the main feature of B-ALL subtype [19] that, due to the differentiation level, can be classified as pro-B, common, precursor B (pre-B), and mature B-cell ALL.

T-ALL is an invasive blood neoplasm characterized by aberrant proliferation of transformed T-cell precursors, and accounts for approximately 15% and 25% of pediatric and adult ALLs, respectively [20 - 22]. The most specific surface marker for lymphoblastic T-cell is represented by CD31, others T-cell markers such as CD1a, and CD2-CD8 are differently expressed and are strictly dependent on the T-cell differentiation degree [23]. A novel subtype of T-cell ALL, ETP T-ALL, has recently been described [24], and is capable to differentiate into both T-cell and myeloid lineages. Indeed, these lineages share high similarities in the myeloid leukemic stem cells gene expression profiles [23]. Concerning the frequency, in children ETP-ALL has been reported to be present in 11% to 16% of T-ALL, while in adults ETP-ALL frequency ranges from 7,4% to 17% of T-ALL [25].

Chromosomal lesions such as translocations are the hallmark of ALL [26 - 28]. Known translocations include t(12;21) [ETV6-RUNX1], also known as TEL-AML1 and found in 22-25% childhood B-ALL [29], t(1;19) [TCF3-PBX1] observed in both adult and pediatric population with an overall frequency of 6% and associated with poor prognosis, t(9;22) [BCR-ABL1] that characterizes the Philadelphia chromosome (Ph) typified by reciprocal translocation of genetic material between chromosome 9 and chromosome 22 and that is frequent in 2% in childhood ALL, with an increment with 50% in the elderly, and t(17; 19) E2A variant translocation occurring in 1% of childhood B-cell precursor ALL cases and responsible of an E2A-HLF (hepatic leukemia factor) fusion gene that induces an aggressive, treatment-resistant pro–B cell stage ALL. In particular, the t(1;19)(q23;p13) TCF3/PBX1 (E2A-PBX1) is also seen in B-ALL (4% of cases). Another translocation involves TAL-1 (SCL) gene (t(1;14)(p34;q11) TAL-1 translocation), with a frequency of nearly 25–30% in T-ALL patients. Aberrant activated SCL during maturation of lymphocytes causes leukemia cells transformation [27, 30 - 32].

The most common genetic rearrangements involve Janus kinase (JAK) mutations, abundantly found in B-ALL subtype and associated with poor prognosis. Activating JAK mutations also correlate with other gene abnormalities, like IKZF1 gene deletion or mutation, that is recurrent from 25 to 30% in B-ALL and at 80% in Ph$^+$ALL, and genomic rearrangement involving the Cytokine receptor-like factor 2 gene (CRLF2) which results in its over expression with poor prognosis [27]. Rearrangements in CRLF2 leads to subsequent B-cell proliferation, and possibly cell transformation, especially in the presence of a constitutively activated JAK mutation. Rearrangements in Platelet Derived Growth Factor Receptor Beta (PDGFRB), in the erythropoietin receptor (EPOR), activating mutations of Interleukin Receptor 7 (IL7R) and deletion of SH2B adapter protein 3 (SH2B3) are also found in B-ALL, especially on the BCR-ABL1–like subtype [33 - 37]. Finally, MLL (mixed-lineage-leukemia) gene rearrangements at 11q23 are also present in 80% of all infant B-ALL cases and 10% of all childhood B-ALL [29].

T-lineage ALL is characterized by activating mutations of Notch1 and other rearrangements, detected in both in pediatric and adult patients [5]. In particular, activating Notch1 mutations, occurring in more than 60% T-ALL, lead to inhibition of ubiquitin mediated degradation of the activated form of Notch1 and are associated with poor prognosis [38].

Current genomic technologies such as Next Generation Sequencing (NGS) or computational genomics, have reported lesions and somatic mutations that can be included into several targetable networks, among which it is necessary to quote

Notch, Jak/Stat, PI3K/Akt/mTOR and MAPK pathways. These pathways are reported to be frequently up-regulated in ALL. Notch1 receptor signaling is involved in T-cell lineage specification, inducing the proliferation of immature T-cell progenitors during lymphogenesis [39]. Relevant Jak/Stat genetic mutations and polymorphisms are significant for different categories of human diseases, including hematologic malignancies [40]. Increased activity of this network is represented in 20-30% of T-ALL. As for MAPK pathway, different genes are frequently dysregulated in ALL cases, including upstream signaling molecules, such as the receptor tyrosine kinase FLT3, or integral components of the pathway such as NRAS and KRAS. In T-ALL and, in addition to these networks, Wnt/β-catenin signaling, chromatin structure modifiers (*i.e.,* KDM6A, CREBBP, EP300, and SMARCB1) and epigenetic regulators that are prevalent in both B-ALL and T-ALL, *i.e.* KMT2D (known as MLL2 in humans and Mll4 in mice), DNMT3A, TET2 or EP300 [41] could open the scenario for a more targeted identification and validation of new genetic biomarkers for better clinical management of ALL.

PI3K/Akt/mTOR Signaling

The phosphoinositide 3-kinase/Akt-signaling pathway is known to be involved in many physiological processes in the cell, including protein synthesis, cell cycle progression, differentiation, metabolism control and apoptosis (Fig. **1**).

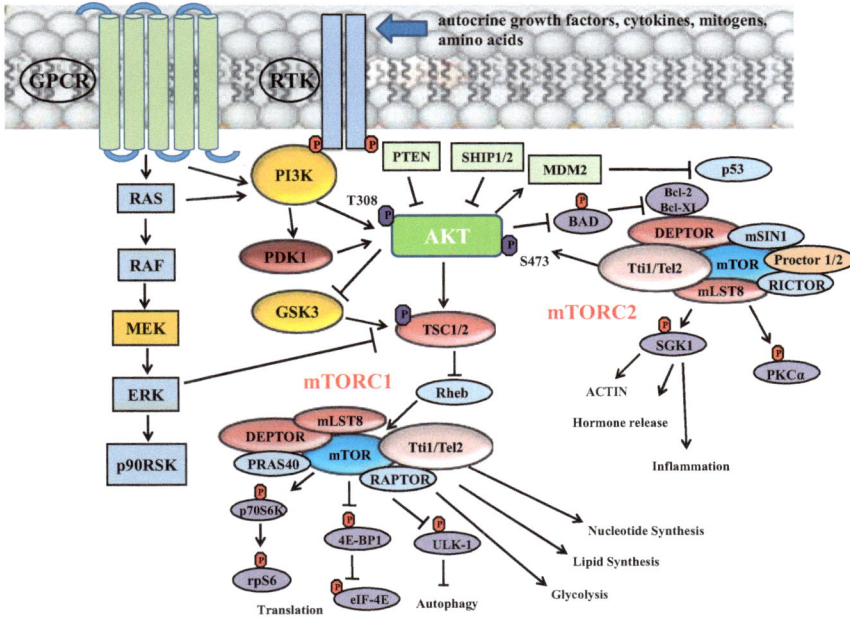

Fig. (1). The PI3K/Akt/mTOR network and the different activities mediated by mTORC1 and mTORC2. The arrows indicate positive interaction, while the T-bars indicate inhibition activity. For the details, see the text.

PI3K is activated by a variety of extracellular stimuli and receptor tyrosine kinases [42] and belongs to a family of lipid kinases that are divided into three classes, of which class I is the most important for oncogenesis. Class I PI3Ks comprises members of a conserved family kinases capable to activate Akt which in turn phosphorylates relevant proteins influencing cell growth and survival. Class IA PI3Ks is composed by a 110 kDa catalytic subunit (p110α, p110β, p110γ, p110δ) and a tightly bound 85 kDa regulatory subunit (p85α, p55α, p50α, p85β, or p55γ). The regulatory subunits maintain the integrity of the catalytic one and direct the heterodimer to membrane associated signaling complexes [43]. Activated PI3K network is controlled by PTEN and loss of activity of this tumor suppressor gene induces an increased downstream activation [44].

PI3K generates the second messenger PtdIns (3,4,5) P3 (PIP3) which recruits Akt and phosphoinositide-dependent protein kinase-1 (PDK1) to the cell membrane. Akt is a 57 kDa serine/threonine protein kinase belonging to the AGC protein kinase family that is activated by phosphorylation by PDK1 at Thr308 and Ser473 [45 - 47]. Akt represents the cellular homolog of the v-akt oncogene [48] with three different isoforms: Akt1/α, Akt2/β, and Akt3/γ. Akt1 and Akt2 are widely expressed in all tissues, while Akt3 is less expressed and therefore limited to some specific tissues, such as brain and testes [49]. Our group was the first to describe the Akt role in the nucleus [50 - 53], and when Akt is present in its phosphorylated form it regulates downstream proteins that control translation and transcription. PIP3 is a substrate of PTEN, that is a dual specificity lipid and protein kinase that counter-regulates the PI3K-dependent signaling by removing the 3-phosphate mainly from PIP3. It functions as a tumor suppressor gene upstream of Akt and it is often mutated, with a consequent activation of several oncogenes, such as TAL1, TLX3 or TLX1 which are believed to represent the clonal T-ALL drivers [54 - 56]. p53 is an apoptosis inducer, and different studies have reported that PI3K/Akt/mTOR hyperactivation is able to inhibit p53-mediated transcription and apoptosis through Mdm2 protein, that acts as a an ubiquitin ligase for p53 [57].

During transcription Akt targets several growth-regulatory transcription factors like FOXO, NFkB, p53, AP1, c-MYC, β-catenin and Hypoxia Inducible Factor-1 (HIF1) that control the expression of pro- and antiapoptotic genes. In particular, the FOXO transcription factors are a subclass of the large forkhead box protein family, predominantly located in the nucleus where they promote transcription of proapoptotic genes. Akt mediated phosphorylation of FOXO masks the nuclear localization signal which leads to nuclear export and proteasomic degradation. The result is inhibition of FOXO's nuclear functions. Akt also regulates the multi-functional Ser and Thr protein kinase glycogen synthase kinase 3 (GSK3), that is composed of two isoforms, GSK3α and GSK3β, with 85% sequence homology.

The nuclear factor kappa B (NFkB) positively regulates cell proliferation, apoptosis and survival [58]. NFkB activity is increased by Akt directly and indirectly: besides direct phosphorylation of NFkB, Akt also phosphorylates and activates IKKα that is responsible for the destruction of the NFkB-Inhibitor IkB.

The mammalian target of rapamycin (mTOR) is a cellular progression regulator and is involved in metabolic mechanisms [59]. This 289-kDa serine/threonine kinase is composed of two separate complexes, mTOR complex 1 (mTORC1) and mTOR complex 2 (mTORC2) [60]. mTORC1 is Rapamycin-sensitive and acts as a survival controller [61], up-regulates the glycolytic pathway with subsequent stimulation of HIF1α [62], regulates the lysosomal function [63] and is involved in the autophagy process in eukaryotic cells [64]. TSC1/TSC2 is a key negative regulator of mTORC1, and it consists of tuberous sclerosis 1 (TSC1) and tuberous sclerosis 2 (TSC2). Akt and extracellular-signal-regulated kinase (ERK1/2) are able to suppress TSC1/2 activity and stimulate mTORC1. Among the different components, mTORC2 is formed by the rapamycin insensitive companion of mTOR (rictor), mSIN1 and Proctor1/2 [65 - 67]. mTORC2 modulates cell migration, metabolism and actin rearrangement, and is involved in regulation of glucose and creatine transporters [61].

Aberrant PI3K/Akt/mTOR Expression in ALL

Aberrant activity of the PI3K/Akt/mTOR network is frequently observed in adult and pediatric B-ALL [68], being associated with poor prognosis in pediatric patients [69, 70]. High expression of mTOR has been demonstrated to correlate with poor clinical outcome in this ALL subtype [71]. Moreover, GSK-3β could act as a negative prognostic indicator in acute leukemias, including pediatric B-ALL [72, 73].

In Ph[+] B-ALL, PI3K activation is dependent on the presence of a multiprotein complex that, besides p110 and p85 PI3K, comprises BCR-ABL and the adaptor proteins, CRKL and c-CRK [74]. The leukemogenic potential of activated PI3K is supported by the evidence that deletion of both *Pik3r1* and *Pik3r2* (which encode for class IA PI3K p85α and p85β, respectively) markedly impaired leukemic transformation. Other models of activation of PI3K in Ph[+] B-ALL have been proposed, including Src family kinases or Ras [75]. Regarding Ph[-] B-ALL, evidence suggests that the aberrant expression of the PI3K/Akt/mTOR pathway could depend on pre-B-cell receptor (pre-BCR) signaling, found in approximately 13% of Ph[-] B-ALL cases, whereas most Ph[-] B-ALL cases lack expression of functional pre-BCR [76].

As to PTEN, both adult Ph[-] and Ph[+] B-ALL primary samples displayed decreased PTEN activity and PI3K/Akt/mTOR network constitutive hyperactivation [77].

Also in this subtype, CK2 activity could be responsible for PTEN post-translational inactivation.

In T-ALL, the constitutively activated PI3K/Akt/mTOR network is mainly due to the inactivation of PTEN [78]. Interestingly, the activation of the PI3K/Akt/mTOR signaling network in normal and malignant thymocytes is correlated to the hematopoietic growth factor IL-7 stimulation [79].

According to the preclinical data, a number of early phase trials are currently open for the analysis of PI3K/Akt/mTOR inhibitors, alone or in combination with conventional therapeutic protocols in hematologic malignancies (see for example www.clinicaltrials.gov), including B- and T-ALL [69, 70, 77, 80, 81].

PI3K Inhibition in ALL

PI3K inhibitors comprise pan p110 PI3K inhibitors and isoform-specific inhibitors. The first report showing that a pan p110 PI3K inhibitor (LY294002) could induce either cell cycle arrest or apoptosis in a Ph⁻ B-ALL cell line, RS4;t11, dates back to 2004 when it was observed that Akt activation was required for the protective effects exerted by human stromal cells on B-ALL cells exposed to chemotherapeutic drugs such as Ara-C and etoposide [82].

LY294002 was able to completely abrogate Interleukin 17A (IL-17A)-mediated protection from daunorubicin-induced apoptosis in B-ALL cells. The cytokine IL-17A normally activates the Akt and Stat3 signaling pathways [83]. Moreover, LY294002 was reported to be cytotoxic and to negatively affect cell growth also in T-ALL cell lines [84, 85].

Among the most recent PI3K inhibitors, BKM-120 (Buparlisib), a pan p110 PI3K inhibitor, showed a significant therapeutic potential. This drug has been tested in the B-ALL subtypes, in cultures of primary Philadelphia positive (Ph⁺) and Philadelphia negative (Ph⁻) B-ALL cells [17], inducing both cell cycle arrest and cell death. More recently, the proapoptotic role of BKM-120 in Ph⁻ B-ALL cells was linked to upregulation of p53-regulated genes [86]. Moreover, it was recently demonstrated to have an acceptable tolerability in a case trial of 14 patients with advanced leukemias (12 affected by acute myeloid leukemia or AML, 1 ALL, and 1 mixed phenotype leukemia), however at 80 mg/day showed modest efficacy [87].

The drug has also been tested in T-ALL models, exerting significant anti-leukemic activity [88, 89]. ZSTK-474, a pan p110 PI3K inhibitor, displayed significant antileukemic effects on three different NUP214-ABL1 positive T-ALL cell lines displaying PI3K/Akt/mTOR activation and showing sensitivity to anti

BCR-ABL1 Tyrosin kinase inhibitors (TKIs) Imatinib, Nilotinib and GZD824. ZSTK-474 alone was cytotoxic, showed inhibition of cellular viability and induced autophagy. The same effects were also detected with the combinations of this drug with the three different TKIs [90]. It was also reported that ZSTK-474 was the most effective in inhibiting the growth of the purine analogue Nelarabine-resistant T-ALL cells and was synergistic with this drug in decreasing survival and inducing apoptosis. Moreover, the drug combination induced Akt dephosphorylation and Bcl2 downregulation [91]. ZSTK-474 displayed important cytotoxic effects also in B-ALL, some of them showing GC-resistance [54, 69].

Besides the pan PI3K inhibitors, the selective PI3K δ/γ inhibitor IPI-145 (Duvelisib) was also partially tested in both in B- and T- ALL, showing anti-leukemic action and inducing apoptosis and autophagy [69, 92].

To overcome the toxicity caused by some pan p110 PI3K inhibitors, novel and selective drugs targeting specifically one or two of the p110 PI3K catalytic subunits have been further tested [93].

CAL-101 (Idelalisib), in Phase I/II clinical trials, is a p110δ PI3K inhibitor accepted in association with rituximab, an anti-CD20 antibody, as a second-line treatment for chronic lymphocytic leukemia (CLL) subjects [94]. CAL-101 has been tested in B-ALL, alone and in association with doxorubicin, exerting G1 blockage (presumably in consequence to up-modulation of p21) and inducing caspase-dependent apoptosis, with subsequent activation of p53 target genes [95].

Importantly, CAL-101 was also able to decrease Akt phosphorylation at Ser 473 on a panel of B-ALL cell lines co-cultured with OP-9 stromal cells, and induced a decreased proliferation when combined with vincristine [96].

To further potentiate the effect of PI3K/Akt/mTOR network inhibition, the development of inhibitors targeting multiple components of the signaling cascade was achieved. These inhibitors, also called dual PI3K/mTOR drugs, have been demonstrated to exert a more powerful anti-leukemic and anti-proliferative effect, and in some cases to promote a greater sensitivity of ALL cells in certain therapeutic protocols, in which the disease was previously resistant. Dual PI3K/mTOR inhibitors interact with ATP-binding sites of mTORC1 and mTORC2, by blocking PI3K/Akt signaling [17, 97]. This class will be discussed in the mTOR inhibition section. A synthesis of the main PI3K inhibitors in B-and T-ALL are reported in Tables **1** and **2**.

Concerning PI3K inhibitors, there is an urgent need to deepen the studies, also in clinical trials, to highlight their effectiveness in the anti-proliferative activity and for the development of new targeted protocols of personalized medicine for ALL treatment. The aim is to offer new therapeutic protocols with the most suitable drug concentrations that can minimize the toxic and collateral effects in all patients.

Table 1. PI3K inhibitors used alone or in association in B-ALL.

Drug Target	Drug	Reported Synergism	Recent Clinical Trials	Reference(s)
pan p110 PI3K	LY294002 (Ph⁻ B-ALL)	-Ara-C -Etoposide -Daunorubicin	No clinical trials are available	[82, 83]
pan p110 PI3K	BKM-120 (Buparlisib) (Ph⁺/ Ph⁻ B-ALL)	-	No clinical trials are available	[86, 87]
pan p110 PI3K	ZSTK-474 (B-ALL)	-	No clinical trials are available	[54, 69]
PI3K δ/γ	IPI-145 (Duvelisib) (B-ALL)	-	No clinical trials are available	[69, 92]
p110δ PI3K	CAL-101 (Idelalisib) (B-ALL)	-Doxorubicin	NCT03742323	[95, 96]

Table 2. PI3K inhibitors used alone or in association in T-ALL.

Drug Target	Drug	Reported Synergism	Recent Clinical Trials	Reference(s)
pan p110 PI3K	LY294002	-	No clinical trials are available	[84, 85]
pan p110 PI3K	BKM-120 (Buparlisib)	-	No clinical trials are available	[-]
pan p110 PI3K	ZSTK-474	-	No clinical trials are available	[90, 91]
PI3K δ/γ	IPI-145 (Duvelisib)	-	No clinical trials are available	[69, 92]

Akt Inhibition

Akt has been reported to be a difficult target to inhibit with ATP-competitive small molecules. Indeed, the ATP-binding pocket of Akt shares many homologies with other members of the AGC kinase family [98]. Despite this, different targeted SMI have been tested. One recent tested Akt inhibitor was Triciribine, that was able also to inhibit DNA synthesis. This inhibitor was only tested in T-ALL models, showing significant antileukemic activity, cytotoxicity, caspase-dependent apoptosis and autophagy [99]. Akt1/Akt2 were significantly dephosphorylated by this drug, that exerted also a good synergism with vincristine, a standard chemotherapeutic drug for treatment of T-ALL patients. There is actually one recruiting clinical trial study regarding the role of this drug in association with the cytosine arabinoside cytarabine (Ara-C) for 40 relapsed ALL patients (NCT02930109). However, the study does not specify the ALL subtype. GSK690693 is an ATP-competitive inhibitor which targets Akt [100] and it has been evaluated in different tumors, including hematologic neoplasms [101 - 103]. GSK690693 was reported to block the growth on a panel of ALL cells, and to induce apoptosis, highlighting the importance of Akt as a target inhibition [101]. Moreover, it has been tested in Ph$^+$ and Ph$^-$ B-ALL cell lines where it induced a cell proliferation block and apoptosis accompanied by a dephosphorylation of Akt downstream targets, including GSK3β, PRAS40 and p70S6K [101]. Importantly, both stimulated peripheral blood CD4$^+$ T-cells from healthy donors and mouse thymocytes were less sensitive to GSK690693 than leukemic cells. Nevertheless, dose-limiting toxicities that are likely on target, associated with hyperglycemia, led to termination of the clinical development of this drug [86].

MK-2206 has also been reported to be a specific Akt inhibitor of considerable importance. It is an orally allosteric drug able to target Akt catalytic and PH domains [104]. Our group demonstrated for the first time the significant cytotoxic activity and the anti-leukemic action of this drug on a panel of T-ALL cells [20]. MK-2206 exerted not only cytotoxic activity to primary T-ALL cells, but also was able to induce programmed cell death in a T-ALL patient cell subset CD34$^+$/CD4$^-$/CD7$^-$. Moreover, MK-2206 has reported to be effective not only when used alone, but also strongly synergized with the mTORC1 inhibitor, RAD001, in both Ph$^-$ B-ALL cell lines and patients [105]. The Akt inhibition was more pronounced in T-ALL cells as a triple simultaneous treatment, that has been shown to have greater efficacy in blocking cells in G0/G1 phase and in inducing both apoptosis and autophagy [106]. Furthermore, in steroid resistant T-ALL cells, methylprednisolone (MP), calcitriol and MK-2206 have a synergistic effect on cellular apoptosis, making MK-2206 an interesting treatment option for steroid resistance in T-ALL [107]. The importance of the overcoming of GC resistance by Akt inhibition has also been emphasized by Piovan *et al* [108]. The group showed that Akt inhibition significantly restores the GC receptor NR3C1 transport to the nucleus and sensitizes T-ALL cells to GC treatments, *in vitro* and *in vivo*.

Another Akt inhibitor that has been tested in ALL, but which is no longer in clinical trial is the alkylphospholipid Perifosine. Perifosine leads to a marked inhibition of Akt phosphorylation by interacting with the pleckstrin homology domain of the kinase, thus preventing Akt membrane localization [109].

A synthesis of the main Akt inhibitors in B- and T-ALL models are reported in Tables **3** and **4**.

Table 3. Akt inhibitors used alone or in association in B-ALL.

Drug Target	Drug	Reported Synergism	Recent Clinical Trials	Reference(s)
Akt	GSK690693 (Ph⁻/ Ph⁻ B-ALL)	-	No clinical trials are available	[101]
Akt	MK-2206 (Ph⁻ B-ALL)	RAD001	NCT01258998	[105]
Akt	Perifosine (B-ALL)	-Daunorubicin	No clinical trials are available	[83, 106, 109]

Table 4. Akt inhibitors used alone or in association in T-ALL.

Drug Target	Drug	Reported Synergism	Recent Clinical Trials	Reference(s)
Akt	GSK690693	-	No clinical trials are available	[86]
Akt	MK-2206	-Methylprednisolone -Calcitriol	NCT01258998	[20, 106 - 108]
Akt	Perifosine	-	No clinical trials are available	[83, 106, 109]

Inherently to the targeted Akt inhibition, other SMIs are under development, therefore the next step will be the approval of their effectiveness, first in preclinical ALL models and subsequently in clinical trials.

Classes of mTOR Inhibitors: Roles of Rapamycin, Rapalogs, Dual PI3K/mTOR Inhibitors and TORKIs

The key activity of mTOR as an Akt regulator, its capability in controlling other signaling pathways such as Notch1 (mainly *via* mTORC2), and its role in directing cell metabolism in healthy and cancer cells led to the development of new targeted and personalized ALL therapies. Three classes of mTOR inhibitors can be described in the context of ALL treatment: allosteric inhibitors [(rapamycin and rapalogs, *i.e.,* RAD001 (everolimus), CCI-779 (temsirolimus)] with mTORC1 as a principal target [110 - 112], the above mentioned ATP-competitive dual PI3K/mTOR drugs [113 - 115] and mTOR kinase inhibitors (TORKIs) that target both mTORC1 and mTORC2, but not PI3K [40, 113, 116].

Rapamycin (Sirolimus) and rapalogs, also known as mTOR first generation inhibitors, report considerable anti-proliferative activity in the clinics, including ALL cases and other types of cancers. Rapamycin is strictly correlated to the intracellular receptor FK506-binding protein 12 (FKBP12), and is involved in the modulation of cytokine signaling inhibition [117].

However, due to some pharmacological limitations, rapamycin has actually been quite outdated, and rapalogs have been subsequently developed for ALL treatment. These rapalogs were known for their minor immunosuppressive activity [117] and greater antitumoral action. As for rapamycin, this class of inhibitors are able to crosslink the immunophilin FK506 binding protein, and induce a dephosphorylation of S6K1 and 4EBP1, with reduction of protein synthesis and a decreased level of cell mortality and size [118]. CCI-779 was the first rapalog to be evaluated for the treatment of different types of cancer, such as breast, non-small-cell lung cancer (NSCLC) and other advanced solid tumors, and in hematological malignancies including ALL [85, 105, 119] exerting anti-proliferative effects, as single agent and in association with rapamycin and other targeted drugs towards signaling pathways different than PI3K/Akt/mTOR. RAD001 has also been investigated for its activity in suppressing tumoral cell growth. It shows a more selective activity for the mTORC1 complex, and it is crucial in inducing caspase-independent and -dependent cell death [120], or in overtaking resistance towards different inhibitors [121].

However, despite the delayed advancement of tumor growth, different studies reported a limited apoptosis induced by rapalogs, and this aspect led to the development of second-generation anti mTOR drugs, that could block the feedback activation of PI3K/Akt pathway and to inhibit both mTOR complexes, bypassing some rapalog limits. As for rapalogs, second-generation anti mTOR drugs reduce protein synthesis and report cytostatic activities, besides inhibiting neo-vascularization in different tumor models [122]. One of the most important advantage of these class is the significant Akt dephosphorylation. Drugs like PKI-587 (Gedatolisib), BEZ235 and BGT226, that are dual PI3K/mTOR inhibitors, have the characteristic of inhibiting mTORC1 and mTORC2 ATP-binding sites, and PI3K catalytic isoforms, with a more pronounced induction of apoptosis and autophagy.

PKI-587, BEZ235 and BGT226 showed significant apoptotic and anti-leukemic activity, and these effects have been reported *in vitro* [17, 90, 123, 124]. Except for BEZ235 that reported one clinical trial study involving 23 refractory ALL patients, PKI-587 and BGT226 have only been tested in vitro. The first inhibitor exhibited a relevant antileukemic effect on ALL, especially on T- leukemia subtype [113] and, in immune-deficient mouse models, delayed the progress of the tumor enhancing the survival rate. The anti-proliferative effect of BEZ235 in ALL cell lines was also documented in different preclinical studies [125, 126], alone and in association with other drugs like GCs, *in vitro* and *in vivo* [126, 127].

An accentuated apoptosis, together with an increased level of the proapoptotic BIM protein, was revealed in PTEN null cells treated with different concentrations of BEZ235 [126, 128]. There are no numerous studies reporting the activity of the dual PI3K/mTOR inhibitor BGT226 on ALL, although it exerted a significant cytotoxic role in the low micromolar range [124] and potently inhibited proliferation inducing cell death in BCR-ABL and TEL-ABL TEL-ABL positive ALL at very low doses [17]. However, the limitation of these inhibitors was an increased toxicity, in different cancer models [122]. Therefore, TORKIs were designed to limit the dual PI3K/mTOR drug toxicity. AZD8055, AZD2014, MLN0128, CC-223, and OSI-027 are examples of TORKIs for the treatment of different solid tumors, such as glioblastoma multiforme, hepatocellular carcinoma, colorectal and pancreatic cancers, but not yet for ALL. Other TORKIs like Ku-0063794 and Torin-2 were tested in B and T-ALL with significant antileukemic activity [17, 90, 123, 129]. However, no clinical trials were reported for these two inhibitors. Further studies are requested to deepen the knowledge for this class of inhibitors, also to overcome some reported resistance mechanisms in solid tumor models, like RTK overexpression/activation or MEK/ERK signaling overactivation [130, 131].

mTOR Inhibition in Ph⁻ B-ALL

B-cell receptor (BCR) is of significant importance both in Ph⁺ B-ALL and also in Ph⁻ B-ALL subtype [132]. BCR signaling characterizes about 13% of Ph⁻ B-ALL cases displaying high expression of B Cell CLL/Lymphoma 6 (BCL6) protein [133], and its activation is strictly dependent on the precursor-B-cell receptor (pre-BCR) stimulated by different inputs that can lead to the activation of aberrant cellular mechanisms in pre-B cells, including a marked and uncontrolled proliferation and tumor invasiveness. Numerous studies reported the apoptotic and anti-leukemic effects of rapamycin also in this subtype, and in *in vivo* models. In REH cells, the association of rapamycin with focal adhesion kinase (FAK) displayed an anti-synergistic effect, further accentuated with a significant cell growth down-regulation, cell cycle blockade and programmed cell death [72]. IL-7 could significantly reverse the antileukemic effects induced by rapamycin, suggesting a crucial aspect of this cytokine in monitoring the mTOR function in B-ALL models, *in vitro* and *in vivo* [134]. CCI-779 inhibitor also reported a marked anti-proliferative activity and apoptosis, both in Ph⁻ B-ALL adult patient lymphoblasts and in NOD/SCID xenograft models, showing peripheral-blood blasts reduction and spleen enlargement [111]. RAD001 inhibitor is also able to exert a good synergism with conventional chemotherapy regimens or other drugs like the proteasome inhibitor bortezomib [135]. RAD001 acts also as an autophagy [136] and caspase-independent apoptosis [137] inducer, and its association with MK-2206 significantly exerts anti-leukemic activity [105]. The importance of this inhibitor was also documented by our research in both Ph⁻ B-ALL cell lines and patients, where RAD001 was tested alone and in association with MK-2206 [104]. BEZ235 has also shown to exert antileukemic effects in Ph⁻ B-ALL cells [124], as well as BTG226 [124]. In Ph⁺ and Ph⁻ primary B-ALL models, BEZ235 synergizes with GX15-070 (Obatoclax), a Bcl-2 inhibitor [138], pointing out a different strategy to check ALL survival. Concerning TORKIs, the cytotoxicity of Torin-2 to a panel of Ph⁻ B-ALL cell lines was recently reported. Torin-2 as a single agent was able to suppress feedback activation of PI3K/Akt, whereas RAD001 needed the combination with MK-2206 to display the same effect [139]. In conclusion, the inhibition of the mTOR pathway is a good therapeutic approach, by using SMI acting at different points of the PI3K/Akt/mTOR cascade, in association with conventional chemotherapy.

mTOR Inhibition in Ph⁺ B-ALL and in Ph-like B-ALL

The introduction of TKIs in Chronic Myeloid Leukemia (CML) and Ph⁺ ALL revolutionized the pharmacological strategies for the treatment of these two subtypes, expanding the possibilities for the development of new therapeutic protocols [140 - 143]. However, survival outcomes still remain at a low level compared to Ph⁻ B-ALL [77]. The combination of Imatinib (IM, first-generation TKI) significantly improved the survival of Ph⁺ ALL, and this was particularly noticed with standard chemotherapy or with allogeneic hematopoietic stem cell transplantation (HSCT) [144 - 146]. The development of second- or third-generation TKI have further documented positive outcomes [147, 148]. In this ALL subtype, the antileukemic activity of mTOR inhibitors acting as single agents is not often enough efficient in bypassing drug-resistance, and therefore the combination with other signaling pathway drugs or with TKI inhibitors is absolutely requested. Targeting the signaling pathway downstream from BCR-ABL, that directly activates mTOR pathway, rapamycin could bypass imatinib resistance in T315I mutation harboring cells. This mutation has been reported to confer resistance to TKIs [149, 150]. mTOR pathway can be aberrantly activated by Imatinib, leading to the onset of relapses. In Ph⁺ B-ALL models, Rapamycin was reported to overcame the imatinib mesylate effect, inducing programmed cell death mechanisms [151]. The ability of RAD001 in overcoming resistance to Imatinib was reported by Kuwatsuka *et al.* in Ph⁺ B-ALL cell subset (CD34⁺/CD38⁻) [121]. The co-administration RAD001/imatinib was more powerful in inducing CD34+/CD38- cell apoptosis than RAD001 as a single agent. Regarding dual PI3K/mTOR drugs, PI-103 and BEZ235 have also been used in Ph⁺ B-ALL pre-clinical models [80]. PI-103 displayed greater effectiveness than rapamycin at suppressing mouse pre-B-ALL and human Ph⁺ B-ALL cells [145]. In Ph⁺ B-ALL nilotinib-resistant cells, the anti-apoptotic MDM2 protein (or human homolog of the murine double minute-2) expression was significantly downregulated after BEZ235 treatment, leading to marked cell death [152]. Concerning TORKIs, the effect of PP242 was mainly seen in Ph$^+$ SUP-B15 cells, where it showed a more pronounced cytotoxic effect and a more significant blockade of mTORC1 activity in association with Imatinib, together with an upregulation of bax and cleaved caspase-3 apoptotic proteins [147]. In preclinical Ph$^-$ and Ph$^+$ pediatric B-ALL, MLN0128 abolished cell growth and increased Dasatinib efficacy, emphasizing the importance of exploring potential applications of this TORKI in the clinics. This inhibitor displayed a low toxicity also in *in vivo* models [153].

A newly identified high-risk B-ALL subtype, frequently found more in adolescents than in adults, is the Philadelphia chromosome-like acute lymphoblastic leukemia (Ph-like ALL). This ALL subtype has adverse clinical features, conferring a poor prognosis [154, 155], and it frequently displays a panel of genetic rearrangements in the cytokine receptor like factor 2 (CLRF2), JAK 1/2/3, FLT3 or platelet-derived growth factor receptor-β (PDGFRB) [156, 157]. These mutations are involved in the PI3K/Akt/mTOR pathway expression modulation, inducing high hyperactivation [155, 158, 159]. The combination of TORKIs with dasatinib was also particularly relevant in ABL-rearranged Ph-like B-ALL, and it was more effective than the administration of the TKI alone, suggesting a rationale, also in the clinics, for testing TKI pharmacological combinations with TORKIs in both pediatric and adult Ph-like B-ALL [140].

A synthesis of the main mTOR drugs in B-ALL are reported in Table **5**.

Table 5. mTOR inhibitors used alone or in association in B-ALL.

Drug Target	Drug/Cells	Reported Synergism	Recent Clinical Trials	Reference(s)
mTORC1	Rapamycin (Sirolimus) (Ph+ B-ALL, Ph- B-ALL, Ph-like B-ALL)	-Imatinib mesylate -Daunorubicin -Focal adhesion kinase (FAK) inhibitor	NCT01184885 NCT00792948	[72, 134, 146, 150 - 152]
mTORC1	CCI-779 (Temsirolimus) (Ph- B-ALL)	-	NCT01614197 NCT01184885 NCT01403415	[111]
mTORC1	RAD001 (Everolimus) (Ph+ B-ALL, Ph- B-ALL)	-Imatinib -Vincristine -Bortezomib -MK2206 -LEE-01 -Glucocorticoids	NCT01523977 NCT00968253 NCT00918333	[71, 104, 105, 120, 121, 135 - 137, 139, 151, 162, 173]

(Table 5) cont.....

Drug Target	Drug/Cells	Reported Synergism	Recent Clinical Trials	Reference(s)
PI3K/mTOR	PI-103 (Ph+ B-ALL)	-Imatinib	No clinical trials are available	[145]
PI3K/mTOR	PKI-587 (Gedatolisib) (Ph+ B-ALL, Ph- B-ALL, Ph-like B-ALL)	-	No clinical trials are available	[113]
PI3K/mTOR	BEZ235 (Ph+ B-ALL, Ph- B-ALL)	-Nilotinib -GX15-070	NCT01756118	[17, 90, 124, 125, 128, 138, 152]
PI3K/mTOR	BGT226 (Ph- B-ALL)	-	No clinical trials are available	[123]
mTORC1/ mTORC2	PP-242 (Ph+ B-ALL)	-	No clinical trials are available	[147]
mTORC1/ mTORC2	Torin-2 (B-pre-ALL)	-MK2206	No clinical trials are available	[139]
mTORC1/ mTORC2	MLN0128 (Ph+ B-ALL, Ph- B-ALL)	-Dasatinib	NCT02484430	[153]

mTOR Inhibition in T-ALL

Numerous studies reported that, in T-ALL, high expression of mTOR was found with greater frequency in adults than in childhood [160].

Rapamycin alone is no longer used today in the treatment of leukemias, and therefore also in T-ALL, but rather it has been replaced by rapalogs such as RAD001 [116], CCI-779 [85], and recently by natural analogues of rapamycin [161]. Pikman *et al.* documented, in *in vitro* and in T-ALL *vivo* models, a good synergism of the CDK4/6 inhibitor LEE-01 (ribociclib) when combined with RAD001 and with GCs, currently employed in the treatment of B- and T-ALL [162]. Aliper and collaborators revealed through bioinformatic analysis different novel drug candidates that could act very similar to rapamycin and metformin, including allantoin and ginsenoside (metformin mimetics), epigallocatechingallate and isoliquiritigenin (rapamycin mimetics), and withaferin A (both). One of the most significant findings was withaferin A compound, that displayed significant pathway- and gene-level similarity to rapamycin. Growing evidence in mouse models and cell-cultures indicated that withaferin A could act as an anti-diabetic, and anticancer agent with potent anti-oxidative, antiinflammatory, anti-proliferative and apoptosis-inducing properties. Moreover, these activities are reported to be mediated through Notch 1 inhibition and mTOR signaling downregulation, with a consequent reduced expression of pS6K and p4E-BP1 [161]. Similarly, also the other compounds reported similar effects, therefore pointing out the potentiality of these natural compounds for future experimental validation.

As for the dual PI3K/mTOR inhibitors, a relevant antileukemic effect of BEZ235 has also been observed in Jurkat and MOLT-4 T-ALL cells, when given in combination with Doxo or GCs [125].

Our group recently demonstrated, in T-ALL, the efficacy of BGT226 in promoting apoptosis, autophagy and PI3K/Akt/mTOR network inhibition, by preserving lymphocyte viability. Indeed, healthy unstimulated T lymphocytes were not influenced by treatments, emphasizing the importance of preserving normal immune function [123].

mTOR inhibitors are also frequently combined with Notch1 signaling network inhibitors. Early uncommitted T-cell precursors that enter the thymus at the cortical-medullary junction express the Notch1 receptor and are exposed to high levels of the Notch ligand Δ-like 4 expressed in the surface of thymic epithelial cells [163]. Dysregulated Notch1 in T-ALL represents one of the most common abnormality, and activates PI3K/AKT/mTOR network at multiple levels [164]. The close interconnection between the two signaling networks is given by the fact that the inhibition of Notch1, that upregulates several PI3K upstream signaling receptors in T-cell progenitors, is strictly correlated with the suppression of mTOR.

The activity of the mTOR inhibitor AZD8055 was analyzed in combination with the BH3-mimetic, ABT-263 (Navitoclax). ABT-263 is an orally active Bcl-2 inhibitor, and it has been tested in Chronic Lymphoid Leukemia (CLL), Non-Hodgkin's Lymphoma and in some solid tumor models like breast cancer, with a limited extent in the context of T-ALL. The combination of AZD8055 with ABT-263 induced a dephosphorylation of 4EBP1 and S6, with a low expression of MCL-1 and a significant tumor regression *in vivo* [165].

Regarding TORKIs, the mTOR inhibitor OSI-027 induced in T-ALL the activation of the proapoptotic BCL2 family member PUMA. In contrast, the mTORC2 activity inhibition and phosphorylation of 4EBP1 resulted in NF κB–mediated expression of the early growth response 1 (EGR1) gene, encoding BIM, a proapoptotic protein. Consequently, T-ALL apoptosis was particularly evident with the interaction of different signaling pathways [166].

A synthesis of the main mTOR inhibitors in T-ALL are reported in Table **6**.

Table 6. mTOR inhibitors used alone or in association in T-ALL.

Drug Target	Drug	Reported Synergism	Recent Clinical Trials	Reference(s)
mTORC1	Rapamycin (Sirolimus)	-Doxorubicin -Cyclophosphamide -Methotrexate	NCT01184885 NCT00792948	[161]
mTORC1	CCI-779 (Temsirolimus)	-	NCT01614197	[85]
mTORC1	RAD001 (Everolimus)	-LEE-01 (ribociclib)	NCT01523977 NCT01184885 NCT00792948 NCT00918333 NCT00968253 NCT03328104	[71, 116, 162, 173]
PI3K/mTOR	PKI-587 (Gedatolisib)	-	No clinical trials are available	[113]
PI3K/mTOR	BEZ235	-Cytarabine (AraC) -Doxorubicin -Glucocorticoids	NCT01756118	[125]
PI3K/mTOR	BGT226	-	No clinical trials are available	[123, 124]
mTORC1/ mTORC2	Torin-2	-	No clinical trials are available	[90]
mTORC1/ mTORC2	OSI-027	-	No clinical trials are available	[166]

Clinical Trials

In the next section the most recent Clinical trial cases concerning the role of the most recent PI3K/Akt/mTOR inhibitors are discussed. The reported trials are mainly in completed status with significant results, in recruiting phase and in active status but not recruiting, except for Akt inhibition, in which clinical studies are only reported in the completed phase.

PI3K Inhibition

Actually few studies related PI3K inhibition are reported in the clinics. The p110δ PI3K inhibitor CAL-101 is in a Phase I recruiting clinical study as a new potential therapeutic alternative for ALL patients with the following characteristics: relapsed, refractory to conventional treatments, and old age. The study involves 24 ALL participants for whom conventional treatments are not recommended. Four increasing doses of CAL-101 are given in four cohorts of six patients each with the primary aim of evaluating the overall response rate and the drug response duration in relapsed adult patients (NCT03742323). The study is ongoing;

therefore, objective outcomes are not yet reported.

In a Phase I clinical study involving 23 adult participants with relapsed or refractory ALL, the dose-limiting toxicity (DLT) of BEZ235 administered twice daily is being evaluated, as well as the assessment of the pharmacodynamic modifications in PI3K/Akt/mTOR pathway (NCT01756118).

To date, no other active clinical studies concerning PI3K inhibition in ALL models are reported. Numerous efforts are therefore required to study new and targeted PI3K inhibitors that could demonstrate significant efficacy in these clinical models, and whose activity has been extensively validated in the preclinical samples.

Akt Inhibition

The most recent Phase 2 study reported the activity profile of the Akt inhibitor MK-2206 in 59 patients affected by relapsed or refractory lymphoma of any histology, and B-ALL. MK-2206 was administered orally for 28 days, and the dose was adjusted based on patient toxicity level. A significant response was observed in 8 (14%) patients (2 complete response and 6 partial response), with median response duration of 5·8 months [167]. In the study it was observed a paradoxical increase of different cytokines, and the outcome was explained by a negative feedback mechanism induced by the Akt inhibitor (NCT01258998).

Currently no other clinical studies are reported concerning the Akt inhibition in the treatment of ALL, therefore also in this case numerous other studies are required to confirm a significant efficacy *in vivo*, after an accurate and deep analysis in preclinical studies of other targeted inhibitors for ALL, such as the Phase 2 Akt inhibitor ARQ 092, currently tested in solid tumors such as hepatocellular carcinoma [168] or the Phase 1/2 Akt inhibitor TIC10, currently used in glioblastoma [169], breast [170], hepatocellular carcinoma [171] or pancreatic cancer [172].

mTOR Inhibition

Among the different clinical trials concerning mTOR inhibition, in an early Phase I pilot study rapamycin was given in combination with Hyper-CVAD (Hyperfractionated Cyclophosphamide, Vincristine, Doxo and Dexamethasone) in B- and T-ALL patients. The purpose of the study was the assessment of the safety and low toxicity of the different drug associations (NCT01614197). In another study, rapamycin is also under study in combination with chemotherapy with or without Donor Stem Cell Transplant in Ph+ B-ALL and T-ALL adults (NCT00792948). In a Phase I/II study, the combination of RAD001 with Hyper-

CVAD high-intensity chemotherapy in relapsed B- or T- ALL patients reduced the phosphorylation of S6 Ribosomal Protein (S6RP), with minor toxicity (NCT00968253) [173]. RAD001 is also tested in combination with the histone deacetylase inhibitor (HDACi) Panobinostat in an active trial involving 124 patients with relapsed multiple myeloma, lymphoma or B- and T-ALL. The combination will help to assess the drug toxicity, as well as the pharmacologic (pharmacokinetic/pharmacodynamic) parameters, and/or biologic aspects (NCT00918333). More than 20 pediatric ALL patients were involved in another Phase I trial study, where RAD001 combination with conventional chemotherapy correlated with minimal residual disease (MRD) (NCT01523977) [71]. In another study enrolling 15 participants affected by T-ALL and T-cell lymphoblastic lymphoma (T-LLy) (NCT03328104) RAD001 is given in a treatment course of 28 days in combination with standard chemotherapy and, among the objectives of the study, the determination of the maximum tolerated dose (MTD), as well as the changes in phosphorylation of Akt and 4EBP1 expression pre- and post RAD001 therapy in peripheral blood mono-nuclear cells (PBMCs) and bone marrow will be assessed.

CCI-779 toxicity in combination with dexamethasone, cyclophosphamide and etoposide is also under analysis in relapsed pediatric ALL and in lymphoma patients. In this trial (NCT01614197) several analytical tests, such as MRD testing lab, will be performed and the effect of CCI-779 on GC resistance and on the mTOR modulation will be investigated.

Regarding TORKIs, MLN0128 in a Phase 2 active clinical trial for 35 relapsed/refractory ALL patients. The study started in October, 2016, is ongoing and enrolled 35 participants. Aims of the study are the determination of CR rate after MLN0128 administration, the overall survival for relapsed/refractory ALL patients and the pro-apoptotic Bim and Puma's expression modulation by the TORKI (NCT02484430).

CONCLUDING REMARKS

PI3K/Akt/mTOR signaling pathway has been clearly proven to be an important survival mechanism and means of treatment resistance in ALL. Different pharmacological and targeted PI3K/Akt/mTOR inhibitors are being tested in ALL preclinical and clinical trials, either as single agents or in association with conventional chemotherapy or other inhibitors directed to different signaling pathways that are reported to be aberrantly expressed or hyperactivated. Assuming that ALL patients have multiple molecular abnormalities, it remains unclear how to determine a hierarchy of aberrations that must be targeted first individually or concurrently to generate optimal antileukemic responses. And this is the challenge: to understand and identify the most indicated inhibitor with significant efficacy and low toxicity for patients affected by this haematological malignancy and in general for the treatment of different cancer types. From the analysis of the clinical trials present today it has emerged that the trials concerning the inhibition of mTOR are in greater number than those focused on the inhibition of PI3K and of Akt, and for this reason different proteomic approaches and computational analysis should provide a more detailed scenario into signal transduction networks, pointing out critical signaling aspects that could lead to the analysis of new potential druggable targets. In addition to the analysis of the intracellular pathways, and in this case of PI3K/Akt/mTOR network, immunotherapeutic or epigenetic approaches could also represent a new treatment strategy for ALL and give a considerable contribution to the progress and consolidation of new pharmacological protocols.

LIST OF ABBREVIATIONS

ALL	Acute lymphoblastic leukemia
(Ph+)	Philadelphia positive
(Ph-)	Philadelphia negative
SMIs	Small Molecule Inhibitors
S6	S6 ribosomal protein
CML	Chronic Myeloid Leukemia
RAS/RAF/MEK/ERK	Ras/Raf/mitogen-activated protein kinase kinase (MEK)/extracellular signal-regulated kinase (ERK)
MRD	Minimal residual disease
HDACi	Histone deacetylase inhibitor
GC	Glucocorticoids
TKIs	Tyrosine Kinase Inhibitors
PTEN	Phosphatase and tensin homolog
EGFR	Epidermal Growth Factor Receptor
pre-B	Precursor B
OS	Overall survival
JAK	Janus kinase
CRLF2	Cytokine receptor-like factor 2 gene
PDGFRB	Platelet Derived Growth Factor Receptor Beta
EPOR	Erythropoietin receptor
IL7R	Interleukin Receptor 7
SH2B3	SH2B adapter protein 3
PDK1	Phosphoinositide-dependent protein kinase-1

HIF-1	Hypoxia Inducible Factor-1
GSK3	Glycogen synthase kinase 3
NFkB	Nuclear factor kappa B
mTOR	Mammalian target of rapamycin
TSC1/TSC2	Tuberous sclerosis 1/2
Rictor	Rapamycin insensitive companion of mTOR
IL-17A	Interleukin 17A
Ara-C	Cytosine arabinoside cytarabine
MP	Methylprednisolone
AML	Acute myelogenous leukemia
FAK	Focal adhesion kinase
HSCT	Hematopoietic stem cell transplantation
IM	Imatinib
CLRF2	Cytokine receptor like factor 2
EGR1	Early growth response 1
DLT	Dose-limiting toxicity
MTD	Maximum tolerated dose
PBMCs	Peripheral blood mono-nuclear cells

CONSENT FOR PUBLICATION

Not applicable.

CONFLICT OF INTEREST

The author confirms that this chapter contents have no conflict of interest.

ACKNOWLEDGEMENTS

This work was supported by current research funds Fondo di Ateneo per la Ricerca Scientifica (FAR) and Fondo per l'Incentivazione alla Ricerca (FIR) (G.Z. and L.M.N), Fondazione Di Bella Onlus (L.M.N.).

REFERENCES

[1]   Omran A, Elimam D, Yin F. MicroRNAs: new insights into chronic childhood diseases. BioMed Res Int 2013; 2013: 291826.
[http://dx.doi.org/10.1155/2013/291826] [PMID: 23878802]

[2]   Almashhrawi AA, Ahmed KT, Rahman RN, Hammoud GM, Ibdah JA. Liver diseases in pregnancy: diseases not unique to pregnancy. World J Gastroenterol 2013; 19(43): 7630-8.
[http://dx.doi.org/10.3748/wjg.v19.i43.7630] [PMID: 24282352]

[3]   Kajdos M, Janas Ł, Kolasa-Zwierzchowska D, Wilczyński JR, Stetkiewicz T. Microvesicles as a potential biomarker of neoplastic diseases and their role in development and progression of neoplasm. Przegl Menopauz 2015; 14(4): 283-91.
[http://dx.doi.org/10.5114/pm.2015.56540] [PMID: 26848301]

[4]   Razis E, Arlin ZA, Ahmed T, *et al.* Incidence and treatment of tumor lysis syndrome in patients with acute leukemia. Acta Haematol 1994; 91(4): 171-4.
[http://dx.doi.org/10.1159/000204328] [PMID: 7976113]

[5]   Mullighan CG. The molecular genetic makeup of acute lymphoblastic leukemia. Hematol-Am Soc Hemat 2012; pp. 389-96.

[6]   Pui CH, Carroll WL, Meshinchi S. Biology, Risk Stratification, and Therapy of Pediatric Acute Leukemias: An Update (vol 29, pg 551, 2011). J Clin Oncol 2011; 29: 4847.
[http://dx.doi.org/10.1200/JCO.2010.30.7405]

[7]   Blaj C, Schmidt EM, Lamprecht S, *et al.* Oncogenic Effects of High MAPK Activity in Colorectal Cancer Mark Progenitor Cells and Persist Irrespective of RAS Mutations. Cancer Res 2017; 77(7): 1763-74.
[http://dx.doi.org/10.1158/0008-5472.CAN-16-2821] [PMID: 28202525]

[8]   Roskoski R Jr. Vascular endothelial growth factor (VEGF) and VEGF receptor inhibitors in the treatment of renal cell carcinomas. Pharmacol Res 2017; 120: 116-32.
[http://dx.doi.org/10.1016/j.phrs.2017.03.010] [PMID: 28330784]

[9]   Abdelaziz A, Vaishampayan U. Cabozantinib for Renal Cell Carcinoma: Current and Future Paradigms. Curr Treat Options Oncol 2017; 18(3): 18.
[http://dx.doi.org/10.1007/s11864-017-0444-6] [PMID: 28286925]

[10]   Abou-Elkacem L, Arns S, Brix G, *et al.* Regorafenib inhibits growth, angiogenesis, and metastasis in a highly aggressive, orthotopic colon cancer model. Mol Cancer Ther 2013; 12(7): 1322-31.
[http://dx.doi.org/10.1158/1535-7163.MCT-12-1162] [PMID: 23619301]

[11]   Miksad RA. Cabozantinib in the treatment of hepatocellular carcinoma. Future Oncol 2017; 13(22): 1915-29.

[12]   Palomero T, Sulis ML, Cortina M, *et al.* Mutational loss of PTEN induces resistance to NOTCH1 inhibition in T-cell leukemia. Nat Med 2007; 13(10): 1203-10.
[http://dx.doi.org/10.1038/nm1636] [PMID: 17873882]

[13]   Barrett D, Brown VI, Grupp SA, Teachey DT. Targeting the PI3K/AKT/mTOR signaling axis in children with hematologic malignancies. Paediatr Drugs 2012; 14(5): 299-316.
[PMID: 22845486]

[14]   Carneiro BA, Kaplan JB, Altman JK, Giles FJ, Platanias LC. Targeting mTOR signaling pathways and related negative feedback loops for the treatment of acute myeloid leukemia. Cancer Biol Ther 2015; 16(5): 648-56.
[http://dx.doi.org/10.1080/15384047.2015.1026510] [PMID: 25801978]

[15]   Chappell WH, Steelman LS, Long JM, *et al.* Ras/Raf/MEK/ERK and PI3K/PTEN/Akt/mTOR inhibitors: rationale and importance to inhibiting these pathways in human health. Oncotarget 2011; 2(3): 135-64.
[http://dx.doi.org/10.18632/oncotarget.240] [PMID: 21411864]

[16]   Georgescu MM. PTEN Tumor Suppressor Network in PI3K-Akt Pathway Control. Genes Cancer 2010; 1(12): 1170-7.
[http://dx.doi.org/10.1177/1947601911407325] [PMID: 21779440]

[17]   Badura S, Tesanovic T, Pfeifer H, *et al.* Differential effects of selective inhibitors targeting the PI3K/AKT/mTOR pathway in acute lymphoblastic leukemia. PLoS One 2013; 8(11): e80070.
[http://dx.doi.org/10.1371/journal.pone.0080070] [PMID: 24244612]

[18]   Terwilliger T, Abdul-Hay M. Acute lymphoblastic leukemia: a comprehensive review and 2017 update. Blood Cancer J 2017; 7(6): e577.
[http://dx.doi.org/10.1038/bcj.2017.53] [PMID: 28665419]

[19]   Purizaca J, Meza I, Pelayo R. Early lymphoid development and microenvironmental cues in B-cell acute lymphoblastic leukemia. Arch Med Res 2012; 43(2): 89-101.
[http://dx.doi.org/10.1016/j.arcmed.2012.03.005] [PMID: 22480783]

[20]   Simioni C, Neri LM, Tabellini G, *et al.* Cytotoxic activity of the novel Akt inhibitor, MK-2206, in T-cell acute lymphoblastic leukemia. Leukemia 2012; 26(11): 2336-42.
[http://dx.doi.org/10.1038/leu.2012.136] [PMID: 22614243]

[21]   Girardi T, Vereecke S, Sulima SO, *et al.* The T-cell leukemia-associated ribosomal RPL10 R98S mutation enhances JAK-STAT signaling. Leukemia 2018; 32(3): 809-19.
[http://dx.doi.org/10.1038/leu.2017.225] [PMID: 28744013]

[22]   Martelli AM, Lonetti A, Buontempo F, *et al.* Targeting signaling pathways in T-cell acute lymphoblastic leukemia initiating cells. Adv Biol Regul 2014; 56: 6-21.
[http://dx.doi.org/10.1016/j.jbior.2014.04.004] [PMID: 24819383]

[23]   Marks DI, Rowntree C. Management of adults with T-cell lymphoblastic leukemia. Blood 2017; 129(9): 1134-42.
[http://dx.doi.org/10.1182/blood-2016-07-692608] [PMID: 28115371]

[24]   Iqbal N, Sharma A, Raina V, *et al.* Poor Response to Standard Chemotherapy in Early T-precursor (ETP)-ALL: A Subtype of T-ALL Associated with Unfavourable Outcome: A Brief Report. Indian J Hematol Blood Transfus 2014; 30(4): 215-8.
[http://dx.doi.org/10.1007/s12288-013-0329-1] [PMID: 25435716]

[25]   Jain N, Lamb AV, O'Brien S, *et al.* Early T-cell precursor acute lymphoblastic leukemia/lymphoma (ETP-ALL/LBL) in adolescents and adults: a high-risk subtype. Blood 2016; 127(15): 1863-9.
[http://dx.doi.org/10.1182/blood-2015-08-661702] [PMID: 26747249]

[26]   Chiaretti S, Gianfelici V, O'Brien SM, Mullighan CG. Advances in the Genetics and Therapy of Acute Lymphoblastic Leukemia. American Society of Clinical Oncology educational book American Society of Clinical Oncology Annual Meeting. 35: e314-22.

[27]   Gowda C, Dovat S. Genetic targets in pediatric acute lymphoblastic leukemia. Adv Exp Med Biol 2013; 779: 327-40.
[http://dx.doi.org/10.1007/978-1-4614-6176-0_15] [PMID: 23288647]

[28]   Vicente C, Schwab C, Broux M, *et al.* Targeted sequencing identifies associations between IL7R-JAK mutations and epigenetic modulators in T-cell acute lymphoblastic leukemia. Haematologica 2015; 100(10): 1301-10.
[http://dx.doi.org/10.3324/haematol.2015.130179] [PMID: 26206799]

[29]   Woo JS, Alberti MO, Tirado CA. Childhood B-acute lymphoblastic leukemia: a genetic update. Exp Hematol Oncol 2014; 3: 16.
[http://dx.doi.org/10.1186/2162-3619-3-16] [PMID: 24949228]

[30]   Mullighan CG, Collins-Underwood JR, Phillips LA, *et al.* Rearrangement of CRLF2 in B-progenitor- and Down syndrome-associated acute lymphoblastic leukemia. Nat Genet 2009; 41(11): 1243-6.
[http://dx.doi.org/10.1038/ng.469] [PMID: 19838194]

[31]   Tirado CA, Shabsovich D, Yeh L, *et al.* A (1;19) translocation involving TCF3-PBX1 fusion within the context of a hyperdiploid karyotype in adult B-ALL: a case report and review of the literature. Biomark Res 2015; 3: 4.
[http://dx.doi.org/10.1186/s40364-015-0029-0] [PMID: 25729575]

[32]   Kang ZJ, Liu YF, Xu LZ, *et al.* The Philadelphia chromosome in leukemogenesis. Chin J Cancer 2016; 35: 48.
[http://dx.doi.org/10.1186/s40880-016-0108-0] [PMID: 27233483]

[33]   Boer JM, den Boer ML. BCR-ABL1-like acute lymphoblastic leukaemia: From bench to bedside. Eur J Cancer 2017; 82: 203-18.
       [http://dx.doi.org/10.1016/j.ejca.2017.06.012] [PMID: 28709134]

[34]   Heilmann AM, Schrock AB, He J, *et al.* Novel PDGFRB fusions in childhood B- and T-acute lymphoblastic leukemia. Leukemia 2017; 31(9): 1989-92.
       [http://dx.doi.org/10.1038/leu.2017.161] [PMID: 28552906]

[35]   Konoplev S, Lu X, Konopleva M, *et al.* CRLF2-Positive B-Cell Acute Lymphoblastic Leukemia in Adult Patients: A Single-Institution Experience. Am J Clin Pathol 2017; 147(4): 357-63.
       [http://dx.doi.org/10.1093/ajcp/aqx005] [PMID: 28340183]

[36]   Sakamoto K, Tanaka S, Tomoyasu C, *et al.* Development of acute lymphoblastic leukemia with IgH-EPOR in a patient with secondary erythrocytosis. Int J Hematol 2016; 104(6): 741-3.
       [http://dx.doi.org/10.1007/s12185-016-2083-2] [PMID: 27544511]

[37]   Tasian SK, Loh ML, Hunger SP. Philadelphia chromosome-like acute lymphoblastic leukemia. Blood 2017; 130(19): 2064-72.
       [http://dx.doi.org/10.1182/blood-2017-06-743252] [PMID: 28972016]

[38]   Iacobucci I, Mulligan CG. Genetic Basis of Acute Lymphoblastic Leukemia. J Clin Oncol 2017; 35(9): 975-83.
       [http://dx.doi.org/10.1200/JCO.2016.70.7836] [PMID: 28297628]

[39]   Tzoneva G, Ferrando AA. Recent advances on NOTCH signaling in T-ALL. Curr Top Microbiol Immunol 2012; 360: 163-82.
       [http://dx.doi.org/10.1007/82_2012_232] [PMID: 22673746]

[40]   Man LM, Morris AL, Keng M. New Therapeutic Strategies in Acute Lymphocytic Leukemia. Curr Hematol Malig Rep 2017; 12(3): 197-206.
       [http://dx.doi.org/10.1007/s11899-017-0380-3] [PMID: 28353016]

[41]   Montaño A, Forero-Castro M, Marchena-Mendoza D, Benito R, Hernández-Rivas JM. New Challenges in Targeting Signaling Pathways in Acute Lymphoblastic Leukemia by NGS Approaches: An Update. Cancers (Basel) 2018; 10(4): 10.
       [http://dx.doi.org/10.3390/cancers10040110] [PMID: 29642462]

[42]   Sanchez VE, Nichols C, Kim HN, Gang EJ, Kim YM. Targeting PI3K Signaling in Acute Lymphoblastic Leukemia. Int J Mol Sci 2019; 20(2): 20.
       [http://dx.doi.org/10.3390/ijms20020412] [PMID: 30669372]

[43]   Fruman DA. Regulatory subunits of class IA PI3K. Curr Top Microbiol Immunol 2010; 346: 225-44.
       [http://dx.doi.org/10.1007/82_2010_39] [PMID: 20563711]

[44]   Engelman JA, Luo J, Cantley LC. The evolution of phosphatidylinositol 3-kinases as regulators of growth and metabolism. Nat Rev Genet 2006; 7(8): 606-19.
       [http://dx.doi.org/10.1038/nrg1879] [PMID: 16847462]

[45]   Bayascas JR, Alessi DR. Regulation of Akt/PKB Ser473 phosphorylation. Mol Cell 2005; 18(2): 143-5.
       [http://dx.doi.org/10.1016/j.molcel.2005.03.020] [PMID: 15837416]

[46]   Toker A, Newton AC. Akt/protein kinase B is regulated by autophosphorylation at the hypothetical PDK-2 site. J Biol Chem 2000; 275(12): 8271-4.
       [http://dx.doi.org/10.1074/jbc.275.12.8271] [PMID: 10722653]

[47]   Vincent EE, Elder DJ, Thomas EC, *et al.* Akt phosphorylation on Thr308 but not on Ser473 correlates with Akt protein kinase activity in human non-small cell lung cancer. Br J Cancer 2011; 104(11): 1755-61.
       [http://dx.doi.org/10.1038/bjc.2011.132] [PMID: 21505451]

[48]   Melão A, Spit M, Cardoso BA, Barata JT. Optimal interleukin-7 receptor-mediated signaling, cell

cycle progression and viability of T-cell acute lymphoblastic leukemia cells rely on casein kinase 2 activity. Haematologica 2016; 101(11): 1368-79.
[http://dx.doi.org/10.3324/haematol.2015.141143] [PMID: 27470599]

[49]   Hers I, Vincent EE, Tavaré JM. Akt signalling in health and disease. Cell Signal 2011; 23(10): 1515-27.
[http://dx.doi.org/10.1016/j.cellsig.2011.05.004] [PMID: 21620960]

[50]   Borgatti P, Martelli AM, Bellacosa A, *et al.* Translocation of Akt/PKB to the nucleus of osteoblast-like MC3T3-E1 cells exposed to proliferative growth factors. FEBS Lett 2000; 477(1-2): 27-32.
[http://dx.doi.org/10.1016/S0014-5793(00)01758-0] [PMID: 10899305]

[51]   Borgatti P, Martelli AM, Tabellini G, Bellacosa A, Capitani S, Neri LM. Threonine 308 phosphorylated form of Akt translocates to the nucleus of PC12 cells under nerve growth factor stimulation and associates with the nuclear matrix protein nucleolin. J Cell Physiol 2003; 196(1): 79-88.
[http://dx.doi.org/10.1002/jcp.10279] [PMID: 12767043]

[52]   Missiroli S, Etro D, Buontempo F, Ye K, Capitani S, Neri LM. Nuclear translocation of active AKT is required for erythroid differentiation in erythropoietin treated K562 erythroleukemia cells. Int J Biochem Cell Biol 2009; 41(3): 570-7.
[http://dx.doi.org/10.1016/j.biocel.2008.07.002] [PMID: 18694847]

[53]   Neri LM, Borgatti P, Capitani S, Martelli AM. The nuclear phosphoinositide 3-kinase/AKT pathway: a new second messenger system. Biochim Biophys Acta 2002; 1584(2-3): 73-80.
[http://dx.doi.org/10.1016/S1388-1981(02)00300-1] [PMID: 12385889]

[54]   Evangelisti C, Cappellini A, Oliveira M, *et al.* Phosphatidylinositol 3-kinase inhibition potentiates glucocorticoid response in B-cell acute lymphoblastic leukemia. J Cell Physiol 2018; 233(3): 1796-811.
[http://dx.doi.org/10.1002/jcp.26135] [PMID: 28777460]

[55]   Mendes RD, Canté-Barrett K, Pieters R, Meijerink JP. The relevance of PTEN-AKT in relation to NOTCH1-directed treatment strategies in T-cell acute lymphoblastic leukemia. Haematologica 2016; 101(9): 1010-7.
[http://dx.doi.org/10.3324/haematol.2016.146381] [PMID: 27582570]

[56]   Mendes RD, Sarmento LM, Canté-Barrett K, *et al.* PTEN microdeletions in T-cell acute lymphoblastic leukemia are caused by illegitimate RAG-mediated recombination events. Blood 2014; 124(4): 567-78.
[http://dx.doi.org/10.1182/blood-2014-03-562751] [PMID: 24904117]

[57]   Ogawara Y, Kishishita S, Obata T, *et al.* Akt enhances Mdm2-mediated ubiquitination and degradation of p53. J Biol Chem 2002; 277(24): 21843-50.
[http://dx.doi.org/10.1074/jbc.M109745200] [PMID: 11923280]

[58]   Davoudi Z, Akbarzadeh A, Rahmatiyamchi M, *et al.* Molecular target therapy of AKT and NF-kB signaling pathways and multidrug resistance by specific cell penetrating inhibitor peptides in HL-60 cells. Asian Pac J Cancer Prev 2014; 15(10): 4353-8.
[http://dx.doi.org/10.7314/APJCP.2014.15.10.4353] [PMID: 24935396]

[59]   Kaur A, Sharma S. Mammalian target of rapamycin (mTOR) as a potential therapeutic target in various diseases. Inflammopharmacology 2017; 25(3): 293-312.
[http://dx.doi.org/10.1007/s10787-017-0336-1] [PMID: 28417246]

[60]   Mirabilii S, Ricciardi MR, Piedimonte M, Gianfelici V, Bianchi MP, Tafuri A. Biological Aspects of mTOR in Leukemia. Int J Mol Sci 2018; 19(8): 19.
[http://dx.doi.org/10.3390/ijms19082396] [PMID: 30110936]

[61]   Simioni C, Martelli AM, Zauli G, Melloni E, Neri LM. Targeting mTOR in Acute Lymphoblastic Leukemia. Cells 2019; 8(2): 8.
[http://dx.doi.org/10.3390/cells8020190] [PMID: 30795552]

[62]	Toschi A, Lee E, Gadir N, Ohh M, Foster DA. Differential dependence of hypoxia-inducible factors 1 alpha and 2 alpha on mTORC1 and mTORC2. J Biol Chem 2008; 283(50): 34495-9.
[http://dx.doi.org/10.1074/jbc.C800170200] [PMID: 18945681]

[63]	Settembre C, Zoncu R, Medina DL, *et al.* A lysosome-to-nucleus signalling mechanism senses and regulates the lysosome *via* mTOR and TFEB. EMBO J 2012; 31(5): 1095-108.
[http://dx.doi.org/10.1038/emboj.2012.32] [PMID: 22343943]

[64]	Klionsky DJ, Abdelmohsen K, Abe A, *et al.* Guidelines for the use and interpretation of assays for monitoring autophagy (3rd edition). Autophagy. 2016; 12: pp. 1-222.

[65]	Hara K, Maruki Y, Long X, *et al.* Raptor, a binding partner of target of rapamycin (TOR), mediates TOR action. Cell 2002; 110(2): 177-89.
[http://dx.doi.org/10.1016/S0092-8674(02)00833-4] [PMID: 12150926]

[66]	Jacinto E, Facchinetti V, Liu D, *et al.* SIN1/MIP1 maintains rictor-mTOR complex integrity and regulates Akt phosphorylation and substrate specificity. Cell 2006; 127(1): 125-37.
[http://dx.doi.org/10.1016/j.cell.2006.08.033] [PMID: 16962653]

[67]	Sancak Y, Thoreen CC, Peterson TR, *et al.* PRAS40 is an insulin-regulated inhibitor of the mTORC1 protein kinase. Mol Cell 2007; 25(6): 903-15.
[http://dx.doi.org/10.1016/j.molcel.2007.03.003] [PMID: 17386266]

[68]	Gomes AM, Soares MV, Ribeiro P, *et al.* Adult B-cell acute lymphoblastic leukemia cells display decreased PTEN activity and constitutive hyperactivation of PI3K/Akt pathway despite high PTEN protein levels. Haematologica 2014; 99(6): 1062-8.
[http://dx.doi.org/10.3324/haematol.2013.096438] [PMID: 24561792]

[69]	Ultimo S, Simioni C, Martelli AM, *et al.* PI3K isoform inhibition associated with anti Bcr-Abl drugs shows *in vitro* increased anti-leukemic activity in Philadelphia chromosome-positive B-acute lymphoblastic leukemia cell lines. Oncotarget 2017; 8(14): 23213-27.
[http://dx.doi.org/10.18632/oncotarget.15542] [PMID: 28390196]

[70]	Zhang Q, Shi C, Han L, *et al.* Inhibition of mTORC1/C2 signaling improves anti-leukemia efficacy of JAK/STAT blockade in *CRLF2* rearranged and/or *JAK* driven Philadelphia chromosome-like acute B-cell lymphoblastic leukemia. Oncotarget 2018; 9(8): 8027-41.
[http://dx.doi.org/10.18632/oncotarget.24261] [PMID: 29487712]

[71]	Place AE, Pikman Y, Stevenson KE, *et al.* Phase I trial of the mTOR inhibitor everolimus in combination with multi-agent chemotherapy in relapsed childhood acute lymphoblastic leukemia. Pediatr Blood Cancer 2018; 65(7): e27062.
[http://dx.doi.org/10.1002/pbc.27062] [PMID: 29603593]

[72]	Shi PJ, Xu LH, Lin KY, Weng WJ, Fang JP. Synergism between the mTOR inhibitor rapamycin and FAK down-regulation in the treatment of acute lymphoblastic leukemia. J Hematol Oncol 2016; 9: 12.
[http://dx.doi.org/10.1186/s13045-016-0241-x] [PMID: 26892465]

[73]	Gentzler RD, Altman JK, Platanias LC. An overview of the mTOR pathway as a target in cancer therapy. Expert Opin Ther Targets 2012; 16(5): 481-9.
[http://dx.doi.org/10.1517/14728222.2012.677439] [PMID: 22494490]

[74]	Shishido T, Akagi T, Chalmers A, *et al.* Crk family adaptor proteins trans-activate c-Abl kinase. Genes Cells 2001; 6(5): 431-40.
[http://dx.doi.org/10.1046/j.1365-2443.2001.00431.x] [PMID: 11380621]

[75]	Kharas MG, Fruman DA. ABL oncogenes and phosphoinositide 3-kinase: mechanism of activation and downstream effectors. Cancer Res 2005; 65(6): 2047-53.
[http://dx.doi.org/10.1158/0008-5472.CAN-04-3888] [PMID: 15781610]

[76]	Köhrer S, Havranek O, Seyfried F, *et al.* Pre-BCR signaling in precursor B-cell acute lymphoblastic leukemia regulates PI3K/AKT, FOXO1 and MYC, and can be targeted by SYK inhibition. Leukemia 2016; 30(6): 1246-54.

[http://dx.doi.org/10.1038/leu.2016.9] [PMID: 26847027]

[77]   Dinner S, Platanias LC. Targeting the mTOR Pathway in Leukemia. J Cell Biochem 2016; 117(8): 1745-52.
[http://dx.doi.org/10.1002/jcb.25559] [PMID: 27018341]

[78]   You D, Xin J, Volk A, *et al.* FAK mediates a compensatory survival signal parallel to PI3K-AKT in PTEN-null T-ALL cells. Cell Rep 2015; 10(12): 2055-68.
[http://dx.doi.org/10.1016/j.celrep.2015.02.056] [PMID: 25801032]

[79]   Silva A, Gírio A, Cebola I, Santos CI, Antunes F, Barata JT. Intracellular reactive oxygen species are essential for PI3K/Akt/mTOR-dependent IL-7-mediated viability of T-cell acute lymphoblastic leukemia cells. Leukemia 2011; 25(6): 960-7.
[http://dx.doi.org/10.1038/leu.2011.56] [PMID: 21455214]

[80]   Simioni C, Martelli AM, Zauli G, *et al.* Targeting the phosphatidylinositol 3-kinase/Akt/mechanistic target of rapamycin signaling pathway in B-lineage acute lymphoblastic leukemia: An update. J Cell Physiol 2018; 233(10): 6440-54.
[http://dx.doi.org/10.1002/jcp.26539] [PMID: 29667769]

[81]   Toosi B, Zaker F, Alikarami F, Kazemi A, Teremmahi Ardestanii M. VS-5584 as a PI3K/mTOR inhibitor enhances apoptotic effects of subtoxic dose arsenic trioxide *via* inhibition of NF-κB activity in B cell precursor-acute lymphoblastic leukemia. Biomed Pharmacother 2018; 102: 428-37.
[http://dx.doi.org/10.1016/j.biopha.2018.03.009] [PMID: 29574283]

[82]   Wang L, Fortney JE, Gibson LF. Stromal cell protection of B-lineage acute lymphoblastic leukemic cells during chemotherapy requires active Akt. Leuk Res 2004; 28(7): 733-42.
[http://dx.doi.org/10.1016/j.leukres.2003.10.033] [PMID: 15158095]

[83]   Bi L, Wu J, Ye A, *et al.* Increased Th17 cells and IL-17A exist in patients with B cell acute lymphoblastic leukemia and promote proliferation and resistance to daunorubicin through activation of Akt signaling. J Transl Med 2016; 14(1): 132.
[http://dx.doi.org/10.1186/s12967-016-0894-9] [PMID: 27176825]

[84]   Chiarini F, Falà F, Tazzari PL, *et al.* Dual inhibition of class IA phosphatidylinositol 3-kinase and mammalian target of rapamycin as a new therapeutic option for T-cell acute lymphoblastic leukemia. Cancer Res 2009; 69(8): 3520-8.
[http://dx.doi.org/10.1158/0008-5472.CAN-08-4884] [PMID: 19351820]

[85]   Batista A, Barata JT, Raderschall E, *et al.* Targeting of active mTOR inhibits primary leukemia T cells and synergizes with cytotoxic drugs and signaling inhibitors. Exp Hematol 2011; 39: 457-72 e3.
[http://dx.doi.org/10.1016/j.exphem.2011.01.005]

[86]   Bashash D, Safaroghli-Azar A, Delshad M, Bayati S, Nooshinfar E, Ghaffari SH. Inhibitor of pan class-I PI3K induces differentially apoptotic pathways in acute leukemia cells: Shedding new light on NVP-BKM120 mechanism of action. Int J Biochem Cell Biol 2016; 79: 308-17.
[http://dx.doi.org/10.1016/j.biocel.2016.09.004] [PMID: 27599915]

[87]   Ragon BK, Kantarjian H, Jabbour E, *et al.* Buparlisib, a PI3K inhibitor, demonstrates acceptable tolerability and preliminary activity in a phase I trial of patients with advanced leukemias. Am J Hematol 2017; 92(1): 7-11.
[http://dx.doi.org/10.1002/ajh.24568] [PMID: 27673440]

[88]   Pereira JK, Machado-Neto JA, Lopes MR, *et al.* Molecular effects of the phosphatidylinositol-3-kinase inhibitor NVP-BKM120 on T and B-cell acute lymphoblastic leukaemia. Eur J Cancer 2015; 51(14): 2076-85.
[http://dx.doi.org/10.1016/j.ejca.2015.07.018] [PMID: 26238016]

[89]   Lonetti A, Antunes IL, Chiarini F, *et al.* Activity of the pan-class I phosphoinositide 3-kinase inhibitor NVP-BKM120 in T-cell acute lymphoblastic leukemia. Leukemia 2014; 28(6): 1196-206.
[http://dx.doi.org/10.1038/leu.2013.369] [PMID: 24310736]

[90]   Simioni C, Ultimo S, Martelli AM, *et al.* Synergistic effects of selective inhibitors targeting the PI3K/AKT/mTOR pathway or NUP214-ABL1 fusion protein in human Acute Lymphoblastic Leukemia. Oncotarget 2016; 7(48): 79842-53.
[http://dx.doi.org/10.18632/oncotarget.13035] [PMID: 27821800]

[91]   Lonetti A, Cappellini A, Bertaina A, *et al.* Improving nelarabine efficacy in T cell acute lymphoblastic leukemia by targeting aberrant PI3K/AKT/mTOR signaling pathway. J Hematol Oncol 2016; 9(1): 114.
[http://dx.doi.org/10.1186/s13045-016-0344-4] [PMID: 27776559]

[92]   Lonetti A, Cappellini A, Spartà AM, *et al.* PI3K pan-inhibition impairs more efficiently proliferation and survival of T-cell acute lymphoblastic leukemia cell lines when compared to isoform-selective PI3K inhibitors. Oncotarget 2015; 6(12): 10399-414.
[http://dx.doi.org/10.18632/oncotarget.3295] [PMID: 25871383]

[93]   Hirsch E, Chiarle R. Calming down T cell acute leukemia. Cancer Cell 2012; 21(4): 449-50.
[http://dx.doi.org/10.1016/j.ccr.2012.03.025] [PMID: 22516253]

[94]   Jones JA, Robak T, Brown JR, *et al.* Efficacy and safety of idelalisib in combination with ofatumumab for previously treated chronic lymphocytic leukaemia: an open-label, randomised phase 3 trial. Lancet Haematol 2017; 4(3): e114-26.
[http://dx.doi.org/10.1016/S2352-3026(17)30019-4] [PMID: 28257752]

[95]   Safaroghli-Azar A, Bashash D, Sadreazami P, Momeny M, Ghaffari SH. PI3K-δ inhibition using CAL-101 exerts apoptotic effects and increases doxorubicin-induced cell death in pre-B-acute lymphoblastic leukemia cells. Anticancer Drugs 2017; 28(4): 436-45.
[http://dx.doi.org/10.1097/CAD.0000000000000477] [PMID: 28125433]

[96]   Adam E, Kim HN, Gang EJ, *et al.* The PI3Kδ inhibitor idelalisib inhibits homing in an *in vitro* and *in vivo* model of B aLL. Cancers (Basel) 2017; 9(9): 9.
[http://dx.doi.org/10.3390/cancers9090121] [PMID: 28891959]

[97]   Soares HP, Ming M, Mellon M, *et al.* Dual PI3K/mTOR inhibitors induce rapid overactivation of the MEK/ERK pathway in human pancreatic cancer cells through suppression of mTORC2. Mol Cancer Ther 2015; 14(4): 1014-23.
[http://dx.doi.org/10.1158/1535-7163.MCT-14-0669] [PMID: 25673820]

[98]   Piekarska A, Sadowska-Klasa A, Libura M, Karabin K, Hellmann A. Successful use of nilotinib in the therapy of a patient with a chemoresistant relapse of BCR-ABL1-like phenotype acute lymphoblastic leukemia. Oncol Res Treat 2018; 41(9): 550-3.
[http://dx.doi.org/10.1159/000490121] [PMID: 30121665]

[99]   Evangelisti C, Ricci F, Tazzari P, *et al.* Preclinical testing of the Akt inhibitor triciribine in T-cell acute lymphoblastic leukemia. J Cell Physiol 2011; 226(3): 822-31.
[http://dx.doi.org/10.1002/jcp.22407] [PMID: 20857426]

[100] Rhodes N, Heerding DA, Duckett DR, *et al.* Characterization of an Akt kinase inhibitor with potent pharmacodynamic and antitumor activity. Cancer Res 2008; 68(7): 2366-74.
[http://dx.doi.org/10.1158/0008-5472.CAN-07-5783] [PMID: 18381444]

[101] Levy DS, Kahana JA, Kumar R. AKT inhibitor, GSK690693, induces growth inhibition and apoptosis in acute lymphoblastic leukemia cell lines. Blood 2009; 113(8): 1723-9.
[http://dx.doi.org/10.1182/blood-2008-02-137737] [PMID: 19064730]

[102] Mori M, Vignaroli G, Cau Y, *et al.* Discovery of 14-3-3 protein-protein interaction inhibitors that sensitize multidrug-resistant cancer cells to doxorubicin and the Akt inhibitor GSK690693. ChemMedChem 2014; 9(5): 973-83.
[http://dx.doi.org/10.1002/cmdc.201400044] [PMID: 24715717]

[103] Pan C, Wang D, Zhang Y, Yu W. MicroRNA-1284 inhibits cell viability and induces apoptosis of ovarian cancer cell line OVCAR3. Oncol Res 2016; 24(6): 429-35.

[http://dx.doi.org/10.3727/096504016X14685034103518] [PMID: 28281963]

[104] Hirai H, Sootome H, Nakatsuru Y, *et al.* MK-2206, an allosteric Akt inhibitor, enhances antitumor efficacy by standard chemotherapeutic agents or molecular targeted drugs *in vitro* and *in vivo*. Mol Cancer Ther 2010; 9(7): 1956-67.
[http://dx.doi.org/10.1158/1535-7163.MCT-09-1012] [PMID: 20571069]

[105] Neri LM, Cani A, Martelli AM, *et al.* Targeting the PI3K/Akt/mTOR signaling pathway in B-precursor acute lymphoblastic leukemia and its therapeutic potential. Leukemia 2014; 28(4): 739-48.
[http://dx.doi.org/10.1038/leu.2013.226] [PMID: 23892718]

[106] Cani A, Simioni C, Martelli AM, *et al.* Triple Akt inhibition as a new therapeutic strategy in T-cell acute lymphoblastic leukemia. Oncotarget 2015; 6(9): 6597-610.
[http://dx.doi.org/10.18632/oncotarget.3260] [PMID: 25788264]

[107] Pistor M, Schrewe L, Haupeltshofer S, *et al.* 1,25-OH$_2$ vitamin D$_3$ and AKT-inhibition increase glucocorticoid induced apoptosis in a model of T-cell acute lymphoblastic leukemia (ALL). Leuk Res Rep 2018; 9: 38-41.
[http://dx.doi.org/10.1016/j.lrr.2018.01.003] [PMID: 29892547]

[108] Piovan E, Yu J, Tosello V, *et al.* Direct reversal of glucocorticoid resistance by AKT inhibition in acute lymphoblastic leukemia. Cancer Cell 2013; 24(6): 766-76.
[http://dx.doi.org/10.1016/j.ccr.2013.10.022] [PMID: 24291004]

[109] Chiarini F, Del Sole M, Mongiorgi S, *et al.* The novel Akt inhibitor, perifosine, induces caspase-dependent apoptosis and downregulates P-glycoprotein expression in multidrug-resistant human T-acute leukemia cells by a JNK-dependent mechanism. Leukemia 2008; 22(6): 1106-16.
[http://dx.doi.org/10.1038/leu.2008.79] [PMID: 18385752]

[110] Steelman LS, Martelli AM, Cocco L, *et al.* The therapeutic potential of mTOR inhibitors in breast cancer. Br J Clin Pharmacol 2016; 82(5): 1189-212.
[http://dx.doi.org/10.1111/bcp.12958] [PMID: 27059645]

[111] Teachey DT, Obzut DA, Cooperman J, *et al.* The mTOR inhibitor CCI-779 induces apoptosis and inhibits growth in preclinical models of primary adult human ALL. Blood 2006; 107(3): 1149-55.
[http://dx.doi.org/10.1182/blood-2005-05-1935] [PMID: 16195324]

[112] Zhelev Z, Ivanova D, Bakalova R, Aoki I, Higashi T. Synergistic cytotoxicity of melatonin and new-generation anticancer drugs against leukemia lymphocytes but not normal lymphocytes. Anticancer Res 2017; 37(1): 149-59.
[http://dx.doi.org/10.21873/anticanres.11300] [PMID: 28011485]

[113] Gazi M, Moharram SA, Marhäll A, Kazi JU. The dual specificity PI3K/mTOR inhibitor PKI-587 displays efficacy against T-cell acute lymphoblastic leukemia (T-ALL). Cancer Lett 2017; 392: 9-16.
[http://dx.doi.org/10.1016/j.canlet.2017.01.035] [PMID: 28159681]

[114] Martelli AM, Chiarini F, Evangelisti C, *et al.* Two hits are better than one: targeting both phosphatidylinositol 3-kinase and mammalian target of rapamycin as a therapeutic strategy for acute leukemia treatment. Oncotarget 2012; 3(4): 371-94.
[http://dx.doi.org/10.18632/oncotarget.477] [PMID: 22564882]

[115] Tasian SK, Teachey DT, Li Y, *et al.* Potent efficacy of combined PI3K/mTOR and JAK or ABL inhibition in murine xenograft models of Ph-like acute lymphoblastic leukemia. Blood 2017; 129(2): 177-87.
[http://dx.doi.org/10.1182/blood-2016-05-707653] [PMID: 27777238]

[116] Carroll WL, Aifantis I, Raetz E. Beating the Clock in T-cell Acute Lymphoblastic Leukemia. Clin Cancer Res 2017; 23(4): 873-5.
[http://dx.doi.org/10.1158/1078-0432.CCR-16-2825] [PMID: 28007775]

[117] Ballou LM, Lin RZ. Rapamycin and mTOR kinase inhibitors. J Chem Biol 2008; 1(1-4): 27-36.
[http://dx.doi.org/10.1007/s12154-008-0003-5] [PMID: 19568796]

[118]   Faivre S, Kroemer G, Raymond E. Current development of mTOR inhibitors as anticancer agents. Nat Rev Drug Discov 2006; 5(8): 671-88.
[http://dx.doi.org/10.1038/nrd2062] [PMID: 16883305]

[119]   Afriansyah A, Hamid AR, Mochtar CA, Umbas R. Targeted therapy for metastatic renal cell carcinoma. Acta Med Indones 2016; 48(4): 335-47.
[PMID: 28143997]

[120]   Saunders PO, Weiss J, Welschinger R, Baraz R, Bradstock KF, Bendall LJ. RAD001 (everolimus) induces dose-dependent changes to cell cycle regulation and modifies the cell cycle response to vincristine. Oncogene 2013; 32(40): 4789-97.
[http://dx.doi.org/10.1038/onc.2012.498] [PMID: 23128395]

[121]   Kuwatsuka Y, Minami M, Minami Y, *et al.* The mTOR inhibitor, everolimus (RAD001), overcomes resistance to imatinib in quiescent Ph-positive acute lymphoblastic leukemia cells. Blood Cancer J 2011; 1(5): e17.
[http://dx.doi.org/10.1038/bcj.2011.16] [PMID: 22829152]

[122]   Zaytseva YY, Valentino JD, Gulhati P, Evers BM. mTOR inhibitors in cancer therapy. Cancer Lett 2012; 319(1): 1-7.
[http://dx.doi.org/10.1016/j.canlet.2012.01.005] [PMID: 22261336]

[123]   Alameen AA, Simioni C, Martelli AM, *et al.* Healthy CD4+ T lymphocytes are not affected by targeted therapies against the PI3K/Akt/mTOR pathway in T-cell acute lymphoblastic leukemia. Oncotarget 2016; 7(34): 55690-703.
[http://dx.doi.org/10.18632/oncotarget.10984] [PMID: 27494886]

[124]   Wong J, Welschinger R, Hewson J, Bradstock KF, Bendall LJ. Efficacy of dual PI-3K and mTOR inhibitors *in vitro* and *in vivo* in acute lymphoblastic leukemia. Oncotarget 2014; 5(21): 10460-72.
[http://dx.doi.org/10.18632/oncotarget.2260] [PMID: 25361005]

[125]   Schult C, Dahlhaus M, Glass A, *et al.* The dual kinase inhibitor NVP-BEZ235 in combination with cytotoxic drugs exerts anti-proliferative activity towards acute lymphoblastic leukemia cells. Anticancer Res 2012; 32(2): 463-74.
[PMID: 22287733]

[126]   Hall CP, Reynolds CP, Kang MH. Modulation of Glucocorticoid Resistance in Pediatric T-cell Acute Lymphoblastic Leukemia by Increasing BIM Expression with the PI3K/mTOR Inhibitor BEZ235. Clin Cancer Res 2016; 22(3): 621-32.
[http://dx.doi.org/10.1158/1078-0432.CCR-15-0114] [PMID: 26080839]

[127]   Li Y, Buijs-Gladdines JG, Canté-Barrett K, *et al.* IL-7 Receptor Mutations and Steroid Resistance in Pediatric T cell Acute Lymphoblastic Leukemia: A Genome Sequencing Study. PLoS Med 2016; 13(12): e1002200.
[http://dx.doi.org/10.1371/journal.pmed.1002200] [PMID: 27997540]

[128]   Reynolds C, Roderick JE, LaBelle JL, *et al.* Repression of BIM mediates survival signaling by MYC and AKT in high-risk T-cell acute lymphoblastic leukemia. Leukemia 2014; 28(9): 1819-27.
[http://dx.doi.org/10.1038/leu.2014.78] [PMID: 24552990]

[129]   Bressanin D, Evangelisti C, Ricci F, *et al.* Harnessing the PI3K/Akt/mTOR pathway in T-cell acute lymphoblastic leukemia: eliminating activity by targeting at different levels. Oncotarget 2012; 3(8): 811-23.
[http://dx.doi.org/10.18632/oncotarget.579] [PMID: 22885370]

[130]   Fujishita T, Kojima Y, Kajino-Sakamoto R, Taketo MM, Aoki M. Tumor microenvironment confers mTOR inhibitor resistance in invasive intestinal adenocarcinoma. Oncogene 2017; 36(46): 6480-9.
[http://dx.doi.org/10.1038/onc.2017.242] [PMID: 28759045]

[131]   Rodrik-Outmezguine VS, Chandarlapaty S, Pagano NC, *et al.* mTOR kinase inhibition causes feedback-dependent biphasic regulation of AKT signaling. Cancer Discov 2011; 1(3): 248-59.

[http://dx.doi.org/10.1158/2159-8290.CD-11-0085] [PMID: 22140653]

[132] Welsh SJ, Churchman ML, Togni M, Mullighan CG, Hagman J. Deregulation of kinase signaling and lymphoid development in EBF1-PDGFRB ALL leukemogenesis. Leukemia 2018; 32(1): 38-48.
[http://dx.doi.org/10.1038/leu.2017.166] [PMID: 28555080]

[133] Ge Z, Zhou X, Gu Y, *et al.* Ikaros regulation of the BCL6/BACH2 axis and its clinical relevance in acute lymphoblastic leukemia. Oncotarget 2017; 8(5): 8022-34.
[http://dx.doi.org/10.18632/oncotarget.14038] [PMID: 28030830]

[134] Brown VI, Fang J, Alcorn K, *et al.* Rapamycin is active against B-precursor leukemia *in vitro* and *in vivo*, an effect that is modulated by IL-7-mediated signaling. Proc Natl Acad Sci USA 2003; 100(25): 15113-8.
[http://dx.doi.org/10.1073/pnas.2436348100] [PMID: 14657335]

[135] Saunders P, Cisterne A, Weiss J, Bradstock KF, Bendall LJ. The mammalian target of rapamycin inhibitor RAD001 (everolimus) synergizes with chemotherapeutic agents, ionizing radiation and proteasome inhibitors in pre-B acute lymphocytic leukemia. Haematologica 2011; 96(1): 69-77.
[http://dx.doi.org/10.3324/haematol.2010.026997] [PMID: 20952516]

[136] Crazzolara R, Bradstock KF, Bendall LJ. RAD001 (Everolimus) induces autophagy in acute lymphoblastic leukemia. Autophagy 2009; 5(5): 727-8.
[http://dx.doi.org/10.4161/auto.5.5.8507] [PMID: 19363300]

[137] Baraz R, Cisterne A, Saunders PO, *et al.* mTOR inhibition by everolimus in childhood acute lymphoblastic leukemia induces caspase-independent cell death. PLoS One 2014; 9(7): e102494.
[http://dx.doi.org/10.1371/journal.pone.0102494] [PMID: 25014496]

[138] Stefanzl G, Berger D, Cerny-Reiterer S, *et al.* The pan-BCL-2-blocker obatoclax (GX15-070) and the PI3-kinase/mTOR-inhibitor BEZ235 produce cooperative growth-inhibitory effects in ALL cells. Oncotarget 2017; 8(40): 67709-22.
[http://dx.doi.org/10.18632/oncotarget.18810] [PMID: 28978065]

[139] Simioni C, Cani A, Martelli AM, *et al.* Activity of the novel mTOR inhibitor Torin-2 in B-precursor acute lymphoblastic leukemia and its therapeutic potential to prevent Akt reactivation. Oncotarget 2014; 5(20): 10034-47.
[http://dx.doi.org/10.18632/oncotarget.2490] [PMID: 25296981]

[140] Gotesman M, Vo TT, Herzog LO, *et al.* mTOR inhibition enhances efficacy of dasatinib in *ABL*-rearranged Ph-like B-ALL. Oncotarget 2018; 9(5): 6562-71.
[http://dx.doi.org/10.18632/oncotarget.24020] [PMID: 29464092]

[141] Müller MC, Cervantes F, Hjorth-Hansen H, *et al.* Ponatinib in chronic myeloid leukemia (CML): Consensus on patient treatment and management from a European expert panel. Crit Rev Oncol Hematol 2017; 120: 52-9.
[http://dx.doi.org/10.1016/j.critrevonc.2017.10.002] [PMID: 29198338]

[142] Shao C, Yang J, Kong Y, *et al.* Overexpression of dominant-negative Ikaros 6 isoform is associated with resistance to TKIs in patients with Philadelphia chromosome positive acute lymphoblastic leukemia. Exp Ther Med 2017; 14(4): 3874-9.
[http://dx.doi.org/10.3892/etm.2017.4941] [PMID: 29042995]

[143] Yang K, Fu LW. Mechanisms of resistance to BCR-ABL TKIs and the therapeutic strategies: A review. Crit Rev Oncol Hematol 2015; 93(3): 277-92.
[http://dx.doi.org/10.1016/j.critrevonc.2014.11.001] [PMID: 25500000]

[144] Dorshkind K, Witte ON. Linking the hematopoietic microenvironment to imatinib-resistant Ph+ B-ALL. Genes Dev 2007; 21(18): 2249-52.
[http://dx.doi.org/10.1101/gad.1600307] [PMID: 17875661]

[145] Kharas MG, Janes MR, Scarfone VM, *et al.* Ablation of PI3K blocks BCR-ABL leukemogenesis in mice, and a dual PI3K/mTOR inhibitor prevents expansion of human BCR-ABL+ leukemia cells. J

Clin Invest 2008; 118(9): 3038-50.
[http://dx.doi.org/10.1172/JCI33337] [PMID: 18704194]

[146] Oliansky DM, Camitta B, Gaynon P, *et al.* Role of cytotoxic therapy with hematopoietic stem cell transplantation in the treatment of pediatric acute lymphoblastic leukemia: update of the 2005 evidence-based review. Biol Blood Marrow Transplant 2012; 18(4): 505-22.
[http://dx.doi.org/10.1016/j.bbmt.2011.12.585] [PMID: 22209888]

[147] Wu JH, Shi FF, Gong YP, Shi R. The mechanism of combination using mTORC1/2 inhibitor and imatinib to suppress cell proliferation of Ph +ALL cell line. Sichuan Da Xue Xue Bao Yi Xue Ban 2017; 48(2): 216-20.
[PMID: 28612529]

[148] Yu G, Chen F, Yin C, *et al.* Upfront treatment with the first and second-generation tyrosine kinase inhibitors in Ph-positive acute lymphoblastic leukemia. Oncotarget 2017; 8(63): 107022-32.
[http://dx.doi.org/10.18632/oncotarget.22206] [PMID: 29291008]

[149] Hirase C, Maeda Y, Takai S, Kanamaru A. Hypersensitivity of Ph-positive lymphoid cell lines to rapamycin: Possible clinical application of mTOR inhibitor. Leuk Res 2009; 33(3): 450-9.
[http://dx.doi.org/10.1016/j.leukres.2008.07.023] [PMID: 18783828]

[150] Short NJ, Kantarjian H, Jabbour E, Ravandi F. Which tyrosine kinase inhibitor should we use to treat Philadelphia chromosome-positive acute lymphoblastic leukemia? Best Pract Res Clin Haematol 2017; 30(3): 193-200.
[http://dx.doi.org/10.1016/j.beha.2017.05.001] [PMID: 29050692]

[151] Yang X, He G, Gong Y, *et al.* Mammalian target of rapamycin inhibitor rapamycin enhances anti-leukemia effect of imatinib on Ph+ acute lymphoblastic leukemia cells. Eur J Haematol 2014; 92(2): 111-20.
[http://dx.doi.org/10.1111/ejh.12202] [PMID: 24112092]

[152] Ding J, Romani J, Zaborski M, *et al.* Inhibition of PI3K/mTOR overcomes nilotinib resistance in BCR-ABL1 positive leukemia cells through translational down-regulation of MDM2. PLoS One 2013; 8(12): e83510.
[http://dx.doi.org/10.1371/journal.pone.0083510] [PMID: 24349524]

[153] Janes MR, Vu C, Mallya S, *et al.* Efficacy of the investigational mTOR kinase inhibitor MLN0128/INK128 in models of B-cell acute lymphoblastic leukemia. Leukemia 2013; 27(3): 586-94.
[http://dx.doi.org/10.1038/leu.2012.276] [PMID: 23090679]

[154] Tran TH, Loh ML. Ph-like acute lymphoblastic leukemia. Hematology (Am Soc Hematol Educ Program) 2016; 2016(1): 561-6.
[http://dx.doi.org/10.1182/asheducation-2016.1.561] [PMID: 27913529]

[155] Kotb A, El Fakih R, Hanbali A, *et al.* Philadelphia-like acute lymphoblastic leukemia: diagnostic dilemma and management perspectives. Exp Hematol 2018; 67: 1-9.
[http://dx.doi.org/10.1016/j.exphem.2018.07.007] [PMID: 30075295]

[156] O'Leary MC, Lu X, Huang Y, *et al.* FDA Approval Summary: Tisagenlecleucel for Treatment of Patients with Relapsed or Refractory B-Cell Precursor Acute Lymphoblastic Leukemia. Clin Cancer Res 2019; 25(4): 1142-6.
[PMID: 30309857]

[157] Kong Y, Wu YL, Song Y, *et al.* Ruxolitinib/nilotinib cotreatment inhibits leukemia-propagating cells in Philadelphia chromosome-positive ALL. J Transl Med 2017; 15(1): 184.
[http://dx.doi.org/10.1186/s12967-017-1286-5] [PMID: 28854975]

[158] Gardner RA, Finney O, Annesley C, *et al.* Intent-to-treat leukemia remission by CD19 CAR T cells of defined formulation and dose in children and young adults. Blood 2017; 129(25): 3322-31.
[PMID: 28408462]

[159] Tian C, Yu Y, Zhang Y. Waldenstrom macroglobulinaemia terminating in acute lymphoblastic

leukaemia after treatment with fludarabine. Br J Hematol 2019; 184: p. (3)322.

[160] Khanna A, Bhushan B, Chauhan PS, Saxena S, Gupta DK, Siraj F. High mTOR expression independently prognosticates poor clinical outcome to induction chemotherapy in acute lymphoblastic leukemia. Clin Exp Med 2018; 18(2): 221-7.
[http://dx.doi.org/10.1007/s10238-017-0478-x] [PMID: 29076004]

[161] Aliper A, Jellen L, Cortese F, *et al.* Towards natural mimetics of metformin and rapamycin. Aging (Albany NY) 2017; 9(11): 2245-68.
[http://dx.doi.org/10.18632/aging.101319] [PMID: 29165314]

[162] Pikman Y, Alexe G, Roti G, *et al.* Synergistic Drug Combinations with a CDK4/6 Inhibitor in T-cell Acute Lymphoblastic Leukemia. Clin Cancer Res 2017; 23(4): 1012-24.
[http://dx.doi.org/10.1158/1078-0432.CCR-15-2869] [PMID: 28151717]

[163] Sanchez-Martin M, Ferrando A. The NOTCH1-MYC highway toward T-cell acute lymphoblastic leukemia. Blood 2017; 129(9): 1124-33.
[http://dx.doi.org/10.1182/blood-2016-09-692582] [PMID: 28115368]

[164] Paganin M, Ferrando A. Molecular pathogenesis and targeted therapies for NOTCH1-induced T-cell acute lymphoblastic leukemia. Blood Rev 2011; 25(2): 83-90.
[http://dx.doi.org/10.1016/j.blre.2010.09.004] [PMID: 20965628]

[165] Dastur A, Choi A, Costa C, *et al.* NOTCH1 represses MCL-1 levels in GSI-resistant T-ALL, making them susceptible to ABT-263. Clin Cancer Res 2019; 25(1): 312-24.
[PMID: 30224339]

[166] Yun S, Vincelette ND, Knorr KL, *et al.* 4EBP1/c-MYC/PUMA and NF-κB/EGR1/BIM pathways underlie cytotoxicity of mTOR dual inhibitors in malignant lymphoid cells. Blood 2016; 127(22): 2711-22.
[http://dx.doi.org/10.1182/blood-2015-02-629485] [PMID: 26917778]

[167] Oki Y, Fanale M, Romaguera J, *et al.* Phase II study of an AKT inhibitor MK2206 in patients with relapsed or refractory lymphoma. Br J Haematol 2015; 171(4): 463-70.
[http://dx.doi.org/10.1111/bjh.13603] [PMID: 26213141]

[168] Roth GS, Macek Jilkova Z, Zeybek Kuyucu A, *et al.* Efficacy of AKT Inhibitor ARQ 092 Compared with Sorafenib in a Cirrhotic Rat Model with Hepatocellular Carcinoma. Mol Cancer Ther 2017; 16(10): 2157-65.
[http://dx.doi.org/10.1158/1535-7163.MCT-16-0602-T] [PMID: 28566435]

[169] Karpel-Massler G, Siegelin MD. TIC10/ONC201-a potential therapeutic in glioblastoma. Transl Cancer Res 2017; 6 (Suppl. 9): S1439-40.
[http://dx.doi.org/10.21037/tcr.2017.10.51] [PMID: 30148071]

[170] Song Y, Lu M, Qiu H, *et al.* Activation of FOXO3a reverses 5-Fluorouracil resistance in human breast cancer cells. Exp Mol Pathol 2018; 105(1): 57-62.
[http://dx.doi.org/10.1016/j.yexmp.2018.05.013] [PMID: 29856982]

[171] Cheng L, Liu YY, Lu PH, *et al.* Identification of DNA-PKcs as a primary resistance factor of TIC10 in hepatocellular carcinoma cells. Oncotarget 2017; 8(17): 28385-94.
[http://dx.doi.org/10.18632/oncotarget.16073] [PMID: 28415690]

[172] Zhang Q, Wang H, Ran L, Zhang Z, Jiang R. The preclinical evaluation of TIC10/ONC201 as an anti-pancreatic cancer agent. Biochem Biophys Res Commun 2016; 476(4): 260-6.
[http://dx.doi.org/10.1016/j.bbrc.2016.05.106] [PMID: 27233611]

[173] Daver N, Boumber Y, Kantarjian H, *et al.* A Phase I/II Study of the mTOR Inhibitor Everolimus in Combination with HyperCVAD Chemotherapy in Patients with Relapsed/Refractory Acute Lymphoblastic Leukemia. Clin Cancer Res 2015; 21(12): 2704-14.
[http://dx.doi.org/10.1158/1078-0432.CCR-14-2888] [PMID: 25724525]

Polymeric Nanomedicines in Treatment of Breast Cancer: Review of Contemporary Research

Farooq Ali Khan[1,#], Md. Rizwanullah[2,#], Ahmad Perwez[3], Mohammad Zaki Ahmad[4] and Javed Ahmad[4,*]

[1] *Sri Indu Institute of Pharmacy, Hyderabad, India*

[2] *Department of Pharmaceutics, School of Pharmaceutical Education and Research, Jamia Hamdard, New Delhi, India*

[3] *Genome Biology Lab, Department of Biosciences, Jamia Millia Islamia, New Delhi, India*

[4] *Department of Pharmaceutics, College of Pharmacy, Najran University, Najran, Kingdom of Saudi Arabia (KSA)*

Abstract: Among various types of cancers, breast cancer is one of the most frequent and major reasons of cancer death among women worldwide. It has the ability to spread to different organs of the body and develop metastases. Till date, chemotherapy is the most common option for the treatment of breast cancer. However, chemotherapy is not a very successful strategy to cure breast cancer and has decreased the survival rates according to the different breast cancer reports. The inability to deliver a specific drug to the target tissue/cell that causes toxicity to the normal healthy tissue/cell is the primary concern in the chemotherapy. Most of the chemotherapeutic drugs used in conventional chemotherapy have low aqueous solubility and high pre-systemic metabolism; therefore, they are biologically less available to the target location and affect normal healthy tissues/cell as well. Since the last decades, the development of nanoparticle technology has opened a new option in the successful treatment of breast cancer due to the various unique advantages offered by this nanoplatform. Among them, polymeric nanomedicines become the promising choice as the effective drug delivery system and provide great potential in the management of breast cancers as per the outcome of different preclinical studies. Polymeric nanomedicines may exhibit their anticancer efficacy either *via* passive or active targeting approach. Polymeric nanomedicines can be actively targeted by its surface conjugation to the breast cancer-specific targeting ligands. Active targeting of the nanomedicines has the ability to deliver the specific drug to the target site, therefore, healthy cells remain unaffected by active targeting. Moreover, polymeric nanomedicines have also been exploited in breast cancer treatment through gene therapy. This chapter summarizes the extensive literature of preclinical findings on polymeric nanomedicines exploited in the treatment of breast cancer.

* **Corresponding author Javed Ahmad:** Department of Pharmaceutics, College of Pharmacy, Najran University, Najran, Kingdom of Saudi Arabia (KSA); Tel: +966-550957371;
E-mail: jahmad18@gmail.com
# These authors contributed equally to this work

Atta-ur-Rahman and M. Iqbal Choudhary (Eds.)

Keywords: Breast Cancer, Chemotherapy, Polymeric Nanomedicine, Targeted Delivery, Ligand, Preclinical Studies.

INTRODUCTION

Human bodies are made up of more than 10^{14} cells, and cancer can begin with one single cell or a group of cells that have mutations in them. The cell division and growth of cells are regulated by signals produced by the cells, and when such signals are faulty, then there is an uncontrolled, unregulated cell growth, which if unchecked by the immune system, leads to the formation of a lump or a tumor. There are more than two hundred types of cancers, classified according to the tissue and cell type of initial tumor. Cancer is known to be the major cause for human death worldwide and is a global pandemic as per the American Cancer Society, and according to the WHO, cancers account for more than 13% of all deaths each year, and this number is expected to reach 45% by 2030. Breast cancer is the most common cancer in women and is the second most common cancer overall. The American Cancer Society estimates about 271,270 new cases and 42,260 deaths in 2019 in the United States alone [1]. Around the globe, it affects more than 2.1 million women every year and is the leading cause of cancer-related deaths in women. Breast tissue consists of fat, duct, connective tissue, and glandular tissue. Breasts develop as a response to estrogens, progesterone, and other hormones such as growth hormone and insulin. Breasts grow mainly during puberty and in lactating women and during pregnancy. Breast cancer is majorly the carcinomas (adenocarcinomas) of epithelial cells lining the milk ducts. Early detection of breast cancer has improved the rate of survival, however, the current mortality rates remain high [2]. While the hallmarks of cancer are many, but from a pharmaceutical science perspective, the challenge is to make the existing few therapies that we have more effective. Chemotherapy remains one of the mainstays in our possible therapies in the fight against cancer. Polymeric nanomedicines are a pragmatic way forward to treat breast cancers as they offer specific targeting to different tumors, modifications and alterations in the nano device.

CHALLENGES IN TREATMENT OF BREAST CANCER

Cancers as such are a complex disease, and amongst different forms of cancers, the breast cancer is a severe complex and heterogeneous disease where there are multiple tumor entities which have different clinical behaviors and have distinct histological patterns. Breast cancers usually metastasize into the lungs, liver, lymph, and brain, a significant number of women lose their lives as a result of metastatic breast cancer. Different types of breast special cancers such as basal-like carcinoma, Mucinous carcinoma, neuroendocrine carcinoma, micropapillary carcinoma, papillary carcinoma, medullary carcinoma, acinic cell carcinoma constitute about 25% of breast cancers. The World Health Organization recognizes the existence of more than 18 different types of invasive breast cancers based on their histological type. Such a complex disease needs a multidisciplinary approach for its treatment and novel targets are being identified in these breast special cancers [3]. Breast cancer is defined based on the expression of receptors such as the HER-2 (Human Epidermal Growth Factor Receptor-2), ER (Estrogen Receptor) and PR (Progesterone Receptor). To target these receptors or any other targets, chemotherapy, hormonal therapy and radiotherapy seem to be a better choice of treatment, however, these are conventional methods which have only been able to kill differentiated cells but not able to completely remove the tumors [4].

Radiotherapy uses a high level of radiation and regresses the tumor growth in combination with chemotherapy and kills cells that are unseen during the surgery, preventing a recurrence. However, due to the high levels of radiation, there can be mild to severe side effects such as itching, peeling, soreness of the skin, loss of sensation in the breast tissue, and at the end of the treatment it may leave the skin weepy and moist [5]. Hormonal therapy, on the other hand, either adds or blocks hormones, female hormones play a role in the development of some breast cancer types mainly the estrogen and the progesterone, and hormonal therapy either lowers the levels of female hormones or completely blocks them thereby, preventing the development and growth of cancer cells. Tamoxifen a SERM (Selective Estrogen Receptor Modulator) has been commonly used in breast cancers since it is an anti-estrogen; it completely blocks the attachment of estrogen on the breast cancer cells' ER receptors. However, there are limitations with Tamoxifen as it increases the chances of resistance and also puts one at the risk of uterine cancer. Other agents which block the estrogen production such as Anastrozole causes bone fractures and joint pain [6].

Conventional dosage forms of chemotherapeutic agents lack selectivity in targeting and also cause cytotoxicity by non-targeted cells. Chemotherapy is given as either adjuvant or neoadjuvant chemotherapy, which is used after surgery to remove undetected breast cancer cells and before surgery to regress the tumors, which can be further removed by lumpectomy. Literature suggests that chemotherapy works best in a combination of different drugs and these come with side-effects such as the increased risk of infections, hair-loss, easy bleeding (because of the lesser number of platelets) mouth sores, nausea, vomiting and loss of appetite [7].

Another major limitation in the treatment of breast cancer is special types of breast cancers which are highly complex such as the basal-like breast cancer and the Triple Negative Breast Cancer (TNBC) [8]. The TNBC lacks any of the three discussed receptors, *i.e.,* HER-2, ER, and PR. The basal-like breast cancer is devoid of any HER-2 receptors and low-levels of expression or absence of ER. Around 12-17% of women suffering from cancer showed Triple-Negative type [9]. This absence of receptors makes them clinically aggressive and also makes chemotherapy ineffective. Treatment also becomes ineffective due to the presence of MDR (Multi Drug Resistance) transporters which are responsible for efflux of chemotherapeutic drugs from the tumors, which reduces the concentration of the chemotherapeutic agents below the effective dose [10].

POTENTIAL OF POLYMERIC NANOMEDICINES IN TREATMENT OF BREAST CANCER

Polymers are assemblies of smaller molecules (monomers) in long chains. Polymeric nanomedicines provide controlled release of chemotherapeutic agents, also providing enhanced efficacy and breaking the multidrug resistance. Different polymeric nanomedicines (Fig. **1**) like polymeric nanoparticles, polymeric micelles, dendrimers, polymer-lipid hybrid nanoparticles majorly use polymer-based nanomedicines for breast cancer. They can also be used to treat TNBC [11]. They have been used in the diagnosis and treatment of breast cancers, and the chemotherapeutic agents can be targeted either actively or passively using polymeric nano-sized systems. Polymeric nanocarriers provide an excellent platform for modifying their surface with different ligands. The surface modification gives the nanocarrier different properties which serve different functions. A typical nanocarrier will have the drug in an encapsulating material with a surface coating of targeting moiety or ligand. Encapsulating materials are usually polymers of biodegradable nature, or dendrimers (tree-like macromolecules with branching tendrils that reach out from a central core). Examples of different surface modifiers include polymers such as polyethylene glycol (PEG), lipids which are stimuli-sensitive, specific ligands, aptamer, antibodies (Trastuzumab, Bevacizumab), folate, transferrin, peptides, *etc*. All these targeting moieties improve the specificity of targeting tumors [12, 13].

Delivery of anti-cancer agents by nanomedicine platform for breast cancer therapy has the following advantages:

- The solubility of hydrophobic drugs is enhanced, *i.e.*, the aqueous solubility of poorly soluble drugs is increased, making them suitable for administration.
- Drugs are accumulated in targeted tissues and cell by surface modification. As a result, the side effects and off-target effects are reduced. Chemotherapeutic agents have side effects and toxicities, such as muscle weakness, immunosuppression and hair loss which, can be reduced using nanomedicine.

- Most of the polymers used in nanoparticle systems are biodegradable, therefore, there is an increase in the biocompatibility of the nanomedicine.
- Nano-based systems improve the pharmacokinetics and biodistribution, which in turn enhances the efficiency of the drug on the tumor [14].

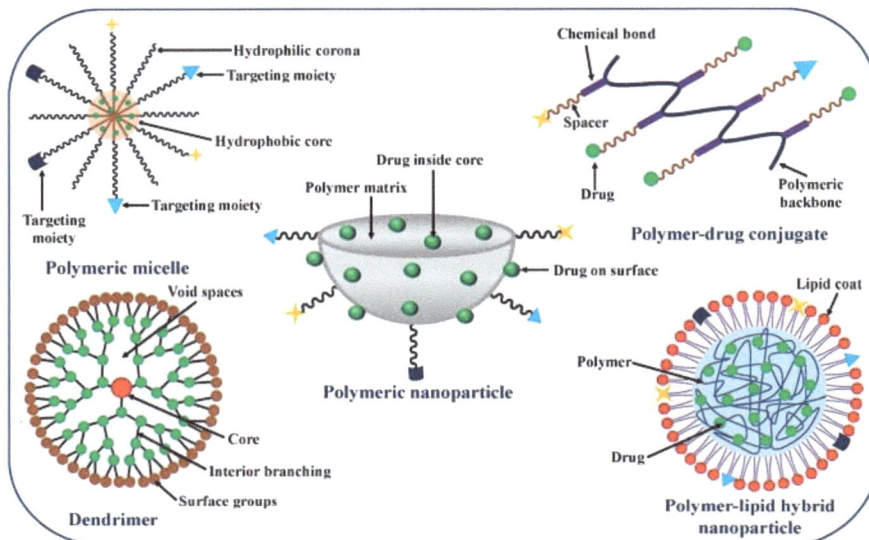

Fig. (1). Different types of polymeric nanomedicines used for chemotherapeutic delivery in the management of breast cancer.

Unprecedentedly in recent years, nanotechnology has been integrated to design new strategies for drug delivery, cell imaging, siRNA and biomedical research. These nanosystems in drug delivery provide a controlled release of the drug which improves the efficacy and helps to overcome drug resistance such systematic and targeted approach to fight disease is presented. In general organic and inorganic nanoparticles are used as drug carriers. Organic systems include polymeric nanoparticles, dendrimers, micelles, carbon nanotubes, liposomes, *etc.* and inorganic nanosystems include gold and silver nanoparticles [15].

The nanocarrier systems can be constructed using an array of materials and can be endowed with special attributes for bioavailability enhancement, targeted delivery to the tumor, gene delivery, combination therapy, theranostic purposes, stimulus-responsive delivery of payload, multimodal anticancer activity, anti-metastatic activity and so on. Nanocarriers can be internalized into tumor cells *via* endocytotic pathways thus evading multidrug resistance (MDR) efflux transporters causing drug resistance [16].

TARGETING IN TREATMENT OF BREAST CANCER

Without special regard to precise delivery to tumors, novel agents in breast cancer will undoubtedly suffer the same fate as traditional chemotherapeutics. Limitations will continue to appear in the form of nonspecific distribution in healthy organs and tissues resulting in toxic side effects, and inadequate accumulation in tumors resulting in reduced efficacy. Targeting of cancer nanomedicine is of two types, passive targeting, and active targeting, as shown in Fig. (**2**).

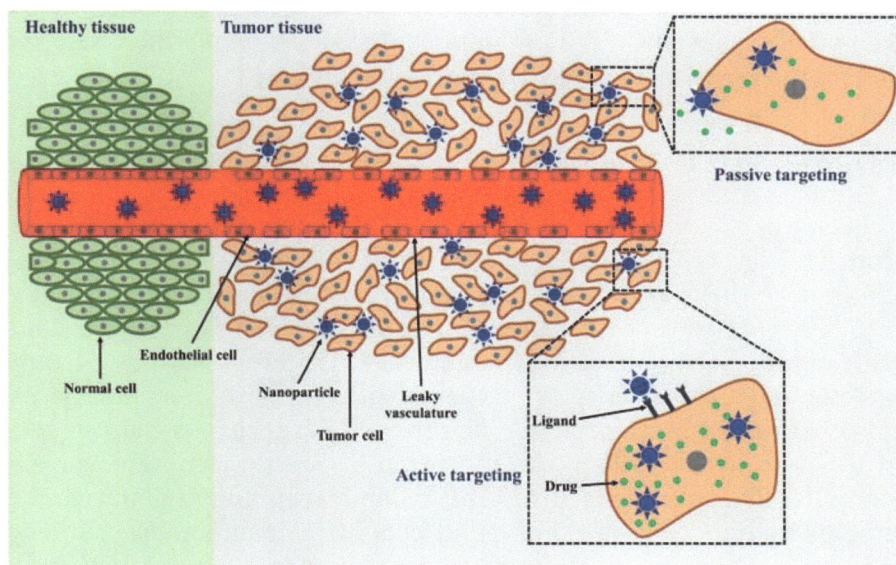

Fig. (2). Passive and active targeting approaches of polymer-based nanomedicines against breast cancer.

Passive Targeting

Passive targeting of nanomedicine to tumors is mainly based on the enhanced permeability and retention (EPR) effect. EPR effect takes into account the two hallmarks of cancer *viz.* the enhanced permeability and the poor lymphatic drainage. Tumors have an ability to form new vasculature, *i.e.*, new blood vessels to meet the blood and nutrient supply to the tumors which are known as angiogenesis, these newly formed blood vessels have enhanced permeability when compared to healthy blood vessels and have poor lymphatic drainage which causes retention of nanomedicine inside the tumors. The pore size in the tumor vasculature is around 100-600 nm when compared to healthy blood vessels which have a pore size of less than 6 nm. Designing of nanomedicine must be made to ensure that it is accumulated in the tumors through the EPR effect and their half-life must be long enough to prevent them from being cleared by the RES (reticuloendothelial system) from the body. The nanomedicine enters the target organ passively and has a therapeutic agent inside it. The EPR effect relies on poor lymphatic drainage of the neovasculature for enhanced retention of the chemotherapeutic agent and the large pores between the adjacent cells in the new blood vessels for improved permeability into the tumors [17].

In case of the passive targeting, the pharmaceutical scientist must focus on controlling the particle size, and the surface of the nanomedicine which will avoid the uptake by RES. The particle size should be below 100 nm which will improve the circulation time and also improve the targeting ability.

Active Targeting

Active targeting of nanomedicine involves the surface modification of decoration or functionalization of the surface with specific ligands or targeting moieties which will bind to the selected tumor site and enable the delivery of drug inside the tumors. This will prevent unwanted side-effects and off-target effects and will enhance the utility of the drug in a better way. Different ligands or targeting moieties which have the affinity for different sites in the tumors can be used to functionalize nanomedicine for active targeting. These ligands help in selective uptake of the drug by having an affinity towards specific receptor expressed on the tumor cells. The enhanced drug uptake and accumulation through active targeting helps to avoid non-target toxic effects of the chemotherapeutic agents. Different receptors have been exploited to actively target tumors, which include the human epidermal growth factor receptor 2 (HER2), EGFR, CD20, transferrin receptor, CD44 receptor, folate receptor, integrin receptor, biotin receptor, *etc.* [4]. The small size of nanomedicine offers a large surface area and presents a large area to bind the ligands specific to tumor cells thereby improving the selective delivery of drugs.

Ligands used in active targeting include aptamers (nucleic acid), antibodies, peptides, *etc.* antibodies are expensive to produce, and their conjugation with the nanomedicine is complicated, but they provide high binding specificity and affinity. Peptides have been used as they have low manufacturing costs compared to antibodies and offer high affinity and targeting specificity. Aptamers have been used because of their low immunogenicity, easy production, and high stability; however, there is a drawback to the use of aptamers as they are a candidate for degradation by nucleases [17].

To improve the active targeting, the pharmaceutical scientist should focus on utilizing overexpressed cell surface receptors on the cancer cells which will help in the internalization of the drug.

DIFFERENT POLYMERIC NANOMEDICINES IN TREATMENT OF BREAST CANCER

Polymers have become an integral part of our daily lives; the word derives its roots from Greek "Poly" meaning many and "Meros" meaning parts or units. Research in polymer science has seen a rapid explosion in recent times because these are versatile materials. Polymers used in drug delivery are usually biodegradable and hence find applicability in biomedical sciences. Polymer-based nanomedicines can overcome various limitations in the current treatment regimen of breast cancer. These systems also have the potential to treat TNBC owing it to their nanosize which can improve the uptake of the drug because of the enhanced permeation and retention (EPR) effect. Several nanomedicine platforms are found to be effective against breast cancer; we focus on polymeric systems which include i.) Polymeric nanoparticles, ii.) Polymeric micelles, iii.) Polymer-lipid hybrid nanoparticles and iv.) Dendrimers.

Polymeric Nanoparticles

Polymeric nanoparticles are matrix-based systems made of polymers having a size in nanometer scale and have been long studied in the field of drug delivery. Nanoparticles have been found to be a powerful platform in breast cancer treatment; currently, nanoparticles of paclitaxel (PTX) and doxorubicin (DOX) are clinically used which explains the potential of this platform. Polymeric nanoparticles offer myriad advantages which include better drug loading, offering control over the drug release, *i.e.*, the release behavior can be adjusted. They also provide an easy surface modification, their industrial scalability is relatively easy, and another significant advantage here is the biodegradability and biocompatibility of polymers. This section will shed light on the current state of research in polymeric nanoparticles designed for breast cancer. In a study, Chen *et al.* developed dual functional nanoparticles of PLGA-PEG for delivery of vincristine sulfate. The nanoparticles were conjugated with folic acid and CPP (Cell-Penetrating Peptide) R7. The system showed a biphasic release of the drug and had a higher cellular uptake when compared to nanoparticles modified only with either of the ligands. Bifunctional conjugation of nanoparticles helped induce a stronger apoptosis and cell cycle arrest in MCF-7 cells which shows that such polymeric nanoparticles have potential in breast cancer management [18]. Choi *et al.* prepared and investigated PLGA nanoparticles for the delivery of Docetaxel.

Herceptin was used as a surface modifier by different techniques such as adsorption, charged adsorption, and bio-conjugation methods. There was a high degree of cellular internalization and strong anti-cancer property of the said nanoparticles in different breast cancer cell lines such as the MCF-7, SK-BR-3, and BT-474 [19]. Cerqueira *et al.* also worked on PLGA nanoparticles of PTX where the surface was coated with hyaluronic acid (HA). HA-grafted PLGA nanoparticles exhibited higher cellular uptake and cytotoxicity against MDA-M--231 cell line based on a possible receptor-mediated endocytosis due to the interaction of HA with CD44 receptors when compared to non targeted PLGA nanoparticles [20]. Talaei *et al.* prepared nanoparticles of thiolated chitosan and tested in T47D breast cancer cells, loading the nanoparticles with DOX and ASOND (Antisense Oligonucleotide), the aim was to study the EGFR effects of the chitosan systems and successfully demonstrated the suppression of EGFR gene expression in the said cancer cell line using ASOND nanoparticles [21]. Dong *et al.* developed mPEG- poly (lactide-coglycolide) (PLGA) nanoparticles for the co-delivery Gemcitabine and PTX to overcome the limitations of systemic toxicity, drug resistance in breast cancer. The cell line studies in MCF-7 and MDA-MB-231 breast cancer cell lines and *in vivo* preclinical studies were carried out in female Balb/C mice which were induced with metastasis-specific mouse mammary carcinoma 4T1 cells to institute breast cancer model. Both *in vitro* and *in vivo* studies have demonstrated that this system has the potential to translate into a safe and effective therapy in the management of breast cancer [22]. Eatemadi *et al.* worked on developing a polymeric nanoparticle system for natural flavonoid Chrysin and studied its effects against breast cancer. Poly(ε-caprolactone) (PCL) and PEG were used to synthesise a triblock co-polymer using ring opening polymerization. They have observed an increase in apoptosis in T47D breast cancer cell line and claim that nanochrysin could be a promising step in breast cancer therapy [23]. In another study carried out by Anari *et al.* Chrysin's effects against breast cancer were evaluated by PLGA-PEG nanoparticles which also demonstrated that nanochrysin in polymeric nanoparticles was effective against T47D cell line [24]. Further, Mishra *et al.* developed Vitamin E TPGS based nanoparticles for Exemestane which were shown to have better antitumor efficacy in MCF-7 breast cancer cells [25]. Ghanghoria *et al.* developed an Luteinizing hormone-releasing hormone (LHRH)-tethered nanoparticle system for PTX delivery and tested the antitumor effects in MCF-7 cells which were the highest when compared to other systems developed by them, the nanoparticle system was also tested in female athymic nude mice with MCF-7 induced tumors and the nanoparticles showed higher tumor uptake and a high degree tumor suppression [26]. Saxena *et al.* targeted folate receptors exploiting nanoparticle system for 17-allylamino-17-demoethoxygeldanamycin which had limitations in clinical due to hepatotoxicity. Studies in MCF-7 breast cancer cells indicated that the formulation had shown higher cytotoxicity and uptake which can be attributed to receptor mediated endocytosis [27]. Hashad *et al.* used HA and human serum albumin as targeting molecules for methotrexate loaded chitosan nanoparticles. 360 kDa HA showed a greater cytotoxicity effect when compared to other grades of HA and human serum albumin. The concentration of targeting moiety used here also played a role in the antitumor effects, and it was stated that 0.1% of working concentration was optimum in preparing different nanoparticles [28]. In another study, Pedro *et al.* developed self-assembled nanoparticles of chitosan to deliver quercetin to breast cancer. Cell line cytotoxicity studies indicate that the quercetin exhibited its inhibition effects against MCF-7 cells after nanoparticle formulation which also could lower its systemic toxicity effects. Internalization of nanoparticles was observed, and even accumulation on the cell membrane was also seen. This system can be used effectively for other hydrophobic drugs as well [29]. Furthermore, Çelebier *et al.* studied the effects of cyclodextrin nanoparticles on MCF-7 cells using biochemical and proteomics, genomics and metabolomics-based investigations [30]. Investigations revealed that non loaded nanoparticles could also trigger different responses in cancer cells when compared to healthy cells. Anionic 6OCaproβCD nanoparticles were found to be a promising approach in passive targeting of cancers.

Summary of different polymeric nanoparticles exploited in the treatment of breast cancer is shown in Table **1**.

Table 1. Polymeric nanoparticles in the treatment of breast cancer.

S. No.	Type of Nanoparticle	Anti-cancer Therapeutics	*In vitro/In vivo* Model	Outcome	Ref.
1	PLGA-PEG bifunctional nanoparticles	Vincristine Sulfate	MCF-7 breast cancer cell line	Strong cell penetration and a higher degree of cytotoxicity and apoptosis in cancer cells.	[18]
2	PLGA nanoparticles	DOX	BT-474, SK-B-3, and MCF-7 breast cancer cell lines	High cell internalization and strong anti-cancer effects in cancer cells and lower cytotoxicity in normal cells.	[19]
3	PLGA nanoparticles	PTX	MDA-MB-231 cell line	Higher cell uptake by receptor-mediated endocytosis	[20]

(Table 1) cont.....

S. No.	Type of Nanoparticle	Anti-cancer Therapeutics	*In vitro/In vivo* Model	Outcome	Ref.
4	N-acetyl cysteine-chitosan nanoparticles and N-acetyl penicillamine-chitosan	DOX and Antisense oligonucleotide	T47D breast cancer cell line	Good cellular uptake and promising downregulation of EGFR expression	[21]
5	mPEG-PLGA nanoparticles	PTX and Gemcitabine	4T1, MCF-7, and MDA-MB-231 cell lines. Female Balb/C mice implanted with 4T1 cancer cells	Reduced cell viability and improved cellular uptake, improved survival time in mice and significant tumor regression, reduced systemic toxicity.	[22]
6	PCL-PEG-PCL triblock copolymer nanoparticles	Chrysin	T47D breast cancer cell line	Increased cytotoxicity and BRCA1 expression, reduced hTERT and FTO gene expression levels, proves a promising approach in breast cancer therapy	[23]
7	PLGA-PEG copolymer nanoparticles	Chrysin	T47D and MCF7 breast cancer cell lines	Higher inhibitory effects.	[24]
8	TPGS-PCL nanoparticles	Exemestane	MCF-7 breast cancer cell line	Enhanced cell uptake and enhanced cytotoxicity.	[25]
9	LHRH-tethered PLGA nanoparticles	PTX	MCF-7 breast cancer cell line, MCF-7-induced tumor female athymic nude mice	High cytotoxicity due to targeting, prolonged circulation, higher tumor uptake and tumor inhibition at low concentrations.	[26]
10	PLGA-PEG nanoparticles	17-allylamino-17-demethoxy geldanamycin (17-AAG)	MCF-7 breast cancer cell line	2 fold increase in the cytotoxicity compared to the free drug.	[27]
11	Chitosan nanoparticles	Methotrexate	MCF-7 breast cancer cell line	Enhanced cancer cell cytotoxicity.	[28]

(Table 1) cont.....

S. No.	Type of Nanoparticle	Anti-cancer Therapeutics	*In vitro/In vivo* Model	Outcome	Ref.
12	Self-assembled chitosan nanoparticles	Quercetin	MCF-7 breast cancer cell line	Quercetin maintains metabolism inhibition activity in the nanoparticle and can reduce side effects.	[29]
13	Cyclodextrin nanoparticles	Amphiphilic cyclodextrin itself	MCF-7 breast cancer cell line	Intrinsic anti-cancer activity of the nanocarrier.	[30]

Polymeric Micelles

Polymeric micelles are colloidal systems which enclose a lipophilic core inside a hydrophilic shell, and the general size of nano-micellar systems ranges from 5 nm to 100 nm. In a study, Greish *et al.* worked on a nano-micellar formulation of a cannabinoid derivative (SMA-WIN) in combination with low doses of DOX. The system showed negligible psychoactive effects, and there was a 60% reduction in tumors in female Balb/c mice with 4T1 mammary carcinoma model. Cell uptake studies in MDA-MB-231, human MCF-7, murine 4T1 cells showed enhanced cytotoxicity. *In vitro* and *in vivo* investigations have shown that it reduced the volume of TNBC murine model drastically [31]. Logie *et al.* docetaxel loaded developed a biodegradable polymeric micelle with a novel taxane-binding peptide (TBP), to overcome the limitations of poor drug loading and poor serum stability generally observed in drug delivery through particulate systems. Taxane binding peptide was used to improve the drug loading of docetaxel as it has the advantage of a new mechanism of known intracellular binding. In comparison with the marketed system, the micellar system had a 2 fold increase in tumor accumulation. The antitumor studies were carried using orthotopic HER2+ breast cancer model in NSG mice. The system showed a proper safety and efficacy profile in the pre-clinical studies making micellar systems a potential area for breast cancer drug delivery [32]. Lu *et al.* developed a dual functional nanomicellar carrier, PEG5Kembelin2 (PEG5K-EB2), which was able to deliver PTX selectively to tumors and to achieve an enhanced therapeutic effect. Based on such a system they investigated the applicability of PEG5K-EB2 in the delivery of DOX. Dual functionality was obtained by coupling folic acid to the micelles along with PEG5K-EB2, to further enhance the selective targeting of the micelles. The size of the drug-loaded micelles was around 20 nm and folic acid functionalization had a negligible effect on the micelles. Folic acid functionalized micelles facilitated the intracellular uptake of DOX as compared to free drug or marketed formulation (Doxil) in 4T1 breast cancer cells. P-gp ATPase assay showed that the micellar formulation inhibited the function of the P-gp efflux pump. The MTD of micelles was 1.5 times higher than the free drug. Their studies further revealed that folic acid functionalized micelles significantly prolonged the plasma circulation of DOX and biodistribution studies indicated that the formulation was preferentially accumulated into the tumors. Tumor regression studies had shown that antitumor activity was increased due to the folic acid functionalization which was higher than free drug and marketed formulation all of which shows micelles as a promising approach for breast cancer management [33]. Further, Mahdaviani *et al.* used a TMT (Tumor metastasis targeting) homing peptide to target drugs to breast cancer cells in conjugation with PEG-PCL micelles for cabazitaxel. Cell line studies were carried out in non-metastatic breast cancer cells (MCF-7) and metastatic breast cancer cells (MDA-MB-231) as well. The tumor necrosis rate was significantly increased, which was almost double due to the targeting by TMT in MDA-MB-231 cell lines. The phenomenon shows that TMT modification can effectively target metastatic breast cancer [34]. Manjili *et al.* developed a curcumin nanomicelles of mPEG-PCL copolymer to target breast cancer. The drug was encapsulated into mPEG-PCL micelles using one step nano-precipitation method. MCF-7 and 4T1 cell lines were used to carry out cytotoxicity studies. *In vivo* pharmacokinetics revealed that the $t_{1/2}$ increased almost 5 times compared to the solution, which indicated prolonged circulation of the drug and improved therapeutic efficacy, and showed that micelles could be a potential system for curcumin delivery to breast cancer [35]. Nosrati *et al.* fabricated biotin-conjugated copolymers based on ring opening polymerization and investigated the micelles by loading artemisinin as cargo. Normal HFF2 cells and breast cancer MCF-7 cells were used for cytotoxicity studies. The micellar formulation was safe on HFF2 cells and had shown the inhibitory effect in MCF-7 breast cancer cells. Tumor suppression studies of the micelles in 4T1 breast cancer model showed a significant reduction in tumor volume when compared to the free drug solution or control group. Drug accumulation had also significantly increased [36]. Guo *et al.* synthesized mPEG-PLGA polymer which was a sensitive to reduction for the co-delivery of docetaxel and a P-gp inhibitor verapamil. Micelles were prepared using this copolymer, which had the ability to overcome MDR and also improve the antitumor effects of docetaxel. The size was around 80 nm, the release was reduction sensitive, and the system had high drug loading, studies also indicated that it inhibited p-gp and improved anticancer effects and reversed MDR [37]. Saxena *et al.* wanted to deliver high concentrations of drug to cancer cells in MDR resistant cancers; They've used vitamin E TPGS and poloxamer 407 to prepare micelles to improve the therapy in MDR resistant tumors. The cargo used in this micellar system was gambogic acid which is a natural novel anticancer molecule with unwanted side effects and poor aqueous solubility. Cellular uptake studies, and other cell line studies were carried out in MCF-7 cells, and multidrug-resistant NCI/ADR-RES cells and the results have shown indicated that drug-loaded poloxamer 407/TPGS mixed micelles had increased cellular uptake in NCI/ADR-RES cells. Higher cytotoxicity was observed, *i.e.,* 1.6 times and suggested that micellar systems can be successfully employed in MDR resistant breast cancers [38]. Qiu *et al.* developed MPEG-PCL micelles to encapsulate luteolin by a self-assembly method, which was aqueous soluble. The micellar formulation significantly improved the pharmacokinetic parameters, and $t_{1/2}$ of luteolin, 4T1 breast cancer cell line studies indicated cytotoxicity and improved anticancer effects [39]. Guzzarlamudi *et al.* prepared micelles of curcumin using a conjugated polymer of mPEG and linoleic acid. The formulation had no hemolytic potential and was highly effective against MCF-7 cells. Cell cycle arrest and apoptosis studies indicated the synergetic effect of micelles and higher apoptosis compared to free drug. $t_{1/2}$ of curcumin was improved which enhanced its retention time. All of the data suggests micelles as a promising approach for breast cancer therapy [40].

Thakur *et al.* developed chitosan-PLGA micelles safe and effective delivery of promising anticancer agent tamoxifen. There was a significant reduction in the IC_{50} values of the drug in MCF-7 cells and also a higher degree of cellular uptake. Dermatokinetic studies in rat skin indicated that the micelles were able to deliver a considerable amount of drug inside the skin when compared to conventional systems [41]. Zhang *et al.* have developed smart micelles, which were to improve the combination of chemo-photothermal therapy. DSPE (1,2-distearoyl-*sn*-glycero-3-phosphoethanolamine-N)- methoxy PEG micelles were selected as a core which encapsulated the drug DOX and these micelles were modified later with PDA (Polydopamine) for photothermal therapy as shell and to deliver bortezomib [42]. The micellar system had a satisfying photothermal efficiency and had the ability to ablate malignant tissues. The system also demonstrated that when combined with laser irradiation it would improve the cytotoxicity and give combinational therapy in MCF-7 tumors and tumor-bearing Balb/c mice with a single nano-sized formulation and could potentially be used as pH-dependent sustained-release and synergized chemo-photothermal therapy of breast cancer [42]. Wang *et al.* developed a pH-dependant micelle-based hydrogels of docetaxel and evaluated for oral delivery. 4T1 breast cancer cell line studies have shown the effective anticancer activity of the micelles; these micelles were incorporated in a pH-sensitive hydrogel. Pharmacokinetic studies indicated that the system had improved the oral bioavailability almost 10 folds when compared to micelles alone, which was due to pH stimuli release of micelles in the small intestine. 4T1 breast cancer model studies indicated that it was effective in inhibiting tumor growth and also reduce toxicities associated with the drug. Apoptosis studies and immunohistochemical studies showed the effectiveness of the formulation and indicated that smart micelle-hydrogel formulation could open new avenues in breast cancer management [43]. In another study, Zhang *et al.* designed PCL-PEG-PCL copolymers in order to overcome toxicities associated with marketed therapy and carried out preclinical investigations [44]. Along with micelles they also designed polymersomes from the same copolymer. The particle size of micelles was 93 nm which was apt for intended IV administration, *in vitro* cytotoxicity demonstrated that the cytotoxic effect of PTX-loaded micelles was lower than that of Taxol. Pharmacokinetic results indicated that the PTX-loaded micelles had longer systemic circulation time and slower plasma elimination rate than those of Taxol. Furthermore, PTX-loaded micelles showed greater tumor growth-inhibition effect *in vivo* on EMT6 breast tumor, in comparison with Taxol.

Summary of different polymeric-drug conjugate/micelles exploited in the treatment of breast cancer is shown in Table **2**.

Table 2. Polymer-drug conjugates/micelles in the treatment of breast cancer.

S. No.	Type of Drug-Conjugate or Micelle	Anti-cancer Therapeutics	*In vitro/In vivo* Model	Outcome	Ref.
1	Poly(styrene-co-maleic anhydride), cumene terminated (SMA) micelles	Cannabinoid derivative, WIN55, 212-2 (WIN) and DOX	MDA-MB-231, 4T1, and MCF-7 breast cancer cell lines. Female Balb/C mice implanted with 4T1 mammary carcinoma tumor	Higher cellular uptake and higher cytotoxicity, higher distribution within tumors, high efficacy, and reduced tumor growth.	[31]
2	Poly(D,L-lactide-co-2-methyl-2-carboxytrimethylene carbonate) (P(LA-co-TMCC)) micelles	Docetaxel	MDA-MB-231/H2N cells, HER2 positive breast cancer tumor in NSG mice	Improved tolerability and long term tumor inhibition.	[32]
3	PEG5K-EB2 micelles	DOX	4T1.2, MCF-7 and NCI/ADR-RES breast cancer cell line, Female BALB/c mice with syngeneic murine breast cancer model (4T1.2)	Effective inhibition and of proliferation, improved cell uptake and accumulation, enhanced tumor inhibition and improved maximum tolerable dose.	[33]
4	PEG-PCL micelles	Cabazitaxel with TMT	MCF-7 and MDA-MB-231 breast cancer cell line	High anti-tumor effects in metastatic MDA-MB-231 cell lines.	[34]
5	mPEG-PCL micelles	Curcumin	MCF-7 and 4T1 breast cancer cell line, BALB/C mice with 4T1 breast cancer model	Remarkable anti-cancer effects, improved systemic circulation and low toxicity to normal cells.	[35]

(Table 2) cont.....

S. No.	Type of Drug-Conjugate or Micelle	Anti-cancer Therapeutics	*In vitro/In vivo* Model	Outcome	Ref.
6	PEG-PCL micelles	Artemisinin	MCF-7 breast cancer cell line, BALB/c mice with 4T1 breast cancer model	High biocompatibility, specific cancer cell cytotoxicity, decreased tumor volumes up to 40 mm^3 than control.	[36]
7	PEG-PLGA conjugate micelles	Docetaxel and verapamil	MCF-7 and MCF-7/ADR breast cancer cell line	Accelerated cell apoptosis, inhibited p-gp efflux, improved tumor inhibition and MDR reversal.	[37]
8	Poloxamer-TPGS mixed micelles	Gambogic acid	MCF-7 and NCI/ADR-RES breast cancer cell line	Increased cellular uptake of cargo in MDR cells, 2.9 times higher cytotoxicity in MDR cells.	[38]
9	Monomethoxy PEG-PCL micelles	Luteolin	4T1 breast cancer cell line	Improved pharmacokinetics, stronger cytotoxicity compared to free drug.	[39]
10	mPEG-Conjugated Linoleic acid micelles	Curcumin	MCF-7 breast cell line	Improved cell-cycle arrest, apoptosis, higher cell uptake and higher breast cancer cell cytotoxicity.	[40]
11	Chitosan-PLGA micelles	Tamoxifen	MCF-7 breast cell line	Enhanced cancer cell cytotoxicity due to improved permeation.	[41]
12	1,2-distearoyl-*sn*-glycero-3-phosphoethanolami-e-N-mPEG (DSPE-mPEG) micelles modified with Polydopamine shell	DOX and Bortezomib	MCF-7 breast cell line, BALB/c athymic nude mice with MCF-7 breast cancer model	Enhanced cytotoxicity, improved chemo-photothermal combinational therapy with synergistic effects against breast cancer.	[42]
13	PEG-PCL micelles based hydrogel	Docetaxel	4T1 breast cancer model	pH-dependent release, efficient inhibition and higher tumor suppression than marketed formulation.	[43]

(Table 2) cont.....

S. No.	Type of Drug-Conjugate or Micelle	Anti-cancer Therapeutics	*In vitro/In vivo* Model	Outcome	Ref.
14	PCL-PEG-PCL triblock polymeric micelles	PTX	EMT6 breast cancer cell line, BALB/c mice with EMT6 breast cancer model	Significant tumor-inhibition, preclinical studies had the potential for clinical studies.	[44]

Polymer-lipid Hybrid Nanoparticles

These are core-shell systems which behave both as nanoparticles and liposomes. Usually, the core is made of polymer, and the shell is made of lipid or lipid-PEG conjugate. These systems overcome the limitations of liposomes and polymeric nanoparticles and provide a robust platform for drug delivery [45]. In a study, Du *et al.* developed a polymer-lipid hybrid nanosystem for delivering psoralen and to enhance its bioavailability and aqueous solubility. The effects of psoralen polymer-lipid hybrid nanoparticles was studied on breast cancer MCF-7 cells and was found efficient with improved antitumor activity and reduced toxicity when compared to DOX, and pharmacokinetic studies revealed that the hybrid carrier system optimized the systemic delivery of psoralen [46]. Tian *et al.* designed a multifunctional nano-sized drug delivery system to deliver antiangiogenic and chemotherapeutic drugs in MDR breast cancer [47]. They developed an amphiphilic material nanoconjugate based on LyP-1 peptide -quercetin conjugate with low molecular weight heparin. They targeted the drug delivery in p32 overexpressing cancer cells and peritumoral lymphatic vessels, LyP1 peptide was used as an active targeting agent and deliver multiple anticancer agents to tumor cells. The functionalization improved the cellular uptake significantly compared to the nonfunctionalized system. The anti-angiogenic activity of lipid-polymer hybrid nanoparticles was effective in inhibiting bFGF-induced neovascularization. High antitumor activity was observed due to inhibition of angiogenesis and cell proliferation with superior targeting ability on p32 overexpressed tumors. More importantly, PLQ/GA nanoparticles with better targeting ability toward p32-positive tumors displayed a high antitumor outcome by inhibition of tumor cells proliferation and angiogenesis. Monirinassab *et al.* hypothesized that polymer-lipid hybrid nanoparticles could deliver siRNA effectively since they have dual advantages and hence developed a PLA-PEG-PLA copolymer using ring-opening polymerization and hybridized it with a cationic lipid by the help of sonication. The system was able to deliver siRNA to tumor cells which were seen in MCF-7 cell line, and down-regulated IGF-1R gene is making this system an effective platform to deliver siRNA to breast cancer [48]. Yang *et al.* optimized and employed a modified emulsification technique to develop polymer-lipid hybrid nanoparticles and investigated the surface properties and stability. They loaded 10-hydroxycampothecin into the system, and the drug release kinetics was not affected by the surface modification. Cytotoxicity and cellular uptake studies in MDA-MB-435s cells have shown that the lipid coverage and the c(RGDyk) conjugation of the hybrid system gave it gained an enhanced ability of endocytosis and cell killing, the data revealed that these systems could be used efficiently deliver drugs to breast cancer cells [49]. In another study, Zhang *et al.* investigated co-delivery of DOX and mitomycin C and find a rationale for co-delivery of drugs, to achieve synergistic effects. The formulation had better biodistribution, improved pharmacokinetics, and reduced toxicity. There was also higher uptake for an extended time which resulted in higher apoptosis and reduced organ toxicities [50]. Furthermore, Zhao *et al.* developed a polymer-core lipid-shell folic acid targeted hybrid Nanoparticulate system to deliver PTX. PLGA was used as core and PEG-OQLCS (PEGylated octadecyl-quaternized lysine modified chitosan) as shell, folic acid as a targeting agent. The hybrid system had shown improved tumor regression in murine models and animal survival upon IV administration. The formulation also had a higher degree of biodistribution in tumors, and this data shows hybrid nanoparticles as a promising approach in cancer therapy [51].

Summary of different polymeric-lipid hybrid system exploited in the treatment of breast cancer is shown in Table **3**.

Table 3. Polymer-lipid hybrid nanosystems in the treatment of breast cancer.

S. No.	Type of Polymer-Lipid Hybrid System	Anti-cancer Therapeutics	*In vitro/In vivo* Model	Outcome	Ref.
1	Phospholipid (Soy Lecithin)-PLGA polymer-lipid nanoparticles	Psoralen	MCF-7 breast cancer cell line, BALB/c mice with MCF-7 cell breast cancer model	Significant tumor growth inhibition, less toxicity against healthy cells.	[46]
2	LyP-1-LMWH nanoparticles	Gambogic acid and Quercetin	MCF-7 breast cancer cell line, BALB/c mice with MCF-7 cell breast cancer model	Higher cell uptake, improved anti-angiogenic activity, dose-dependent cytotoxicity, and improved tumor accumulation.	[47]
3	PLA-PEG-PLA copolymer hybridized with dioctadecyl-ammonium bromide (DDAB Cationic lipid) Hybrid Lipid Nanoparticles	siRNA	MCF-7 breast cancer cell line	Improved intracellular uptake, decrease in IGF-1R expression (Gene silencing).	[48]

(Table 3) cont.....

S. No.	Type of Polymer-Lipid Hybrid System	Anti-cancer Therapeutics	*In vitro/In vivo* Model	Outcome	Ref.
4	DSPE-PEG-PLGA hybrid Lipid Nanoparticles	10-hydroxycamptothecin	MDA-MB-435s breast cancer cell line	Specific targeting and increased cytotoxicity and cell uptake.	[49]
5	PEG100 stearate, PEG40 Stearate and HPESO polymer-lipid nanoparticles	DOX and Mitomycin C	Orthotopic breast tumor model mice with EMT6/WT murine breast cancer cells	Spatiotemporal delivery, improved pharmacokinetics, higher apoptosis in breast tumors.	[50]
6	PLGA- PEGylated octadecyl-quaternized lysine modified chitosan mixed lipid-shell and polymer-core nanoparticles	PTX	Hela cells, SCID mice with Hela cells	High biodistribution, high endocytosis and cytotoxicity in cancer cells.	[51]

Dendrimers

Dendrimers are synthetic macromolecular structures of nanosize usually 10-100 nm which have repetitive units of monomers. These units are arranged as they're emerging from a central core radially. These offer high membrane permeability and target oriented controlled release of the cargo. In a study, Pan *et al.* used a fourth generation poly(amidoamine) (PAMAM) dendrimer-based nanosystem to co-deliver siRNA and DOX in MDR resistant breast cancers [52]. Co-loading of DOX and siRNA was done in the lipidic core, and it was further evaluated for cytotoxicity in MDR cancer cels and MCF-7 cells. The combination of drugs in the micellar system down regulated P-gp in MDR cancer cells effectively and also reversed the resistance towards DOX. Abdel-Rahman *et al.* investigated three thermoresponsive dendrimers based on oligoethylene glycols [53]. The dendrimers were synthesized from tetrabromohydroquinone three different oligoethylene glycol derivatives effectively which had aqueous solubility at room temperature, visually. Cytotoxicity studies of the developed dendrimers were carried out in MCF-7 breast cancer cells, and they've shown considerable results and the second dendrimer gave best results compared to the other two. Bielawski *et al.* evaluated the cytotoxicity of generation 3 PAMAM-NH$_2$ dendrimer which was conjugated with chlorambucil in human breast cancer cell lines, *i.e.*, MDA-MB-231 and MCF-7 [54]. Concentration-dependent growth inhibition was observed in both cell lines; the dendrimer conjugate had higher toxicity when compared to chlorambucil alone. The dendrimer conjugate was more potent and had shown a higher inhibition of collagen biosynthesis and increased apoptosis and necrosis when compared to chlorambucil alone. Chittasupho *et al.* developed a CXCR4 targeted dendrimer and studied effects against breast cancer cells [55]. CXCR4 and its ligand CXCL12 are involved in breast cancer metastasis to lymph nodes, lungs, and bones. LFC131 peptide was conjugated to a generation 4 PAMAM dendrimer by a carbodiimide reaction and was characterized using NMR. DOX was encapsulated directly as a free base using an aqueous solution. DOX generation 4 LFC131 conjugated dendrimers were then studied against BT-549-Luc and T47D breast cancer cell lines for their cell binding, cytotoxicity, and migration. LFC131 recognizes and binds to CXCR4 which is expressed on the metastatic breast cancer cells, and the dendrimer conjugate had shown to enhance the cell binding, improved cytotoxicity significantly when compared to non-conjugated dendrimers. Chemotaxis assays in 24 well migration chamber showed a remarkable reduction of BT-549-Luc cell migration proving LFC131-D4 dendrimer conjugates effective against breast cancer metastasis. Zhao *et al.* prepared a generation 4 PAMAM dendrimer and complexed the dendrimer with VEGF-antisense oligodeoxynucleotides [56]. Breast cancer MDA-MB-231 cell line studies demonstrated that the dendrimer could be used to deliver oligonucleotides without any normal cell toxicity and also improved the cell uptake of oligonucleotides. *In vivo* studies were carried out in human breast tumor xenograft mice model, and the generation 4 dendrimer demonstrated efficient accumulation of VEGF-antisense oligodeoxynucleotides into tumor vasculature when compared to naked antisense oligodeoxynucleotides. Kulhari *et al.* synthesized trastuzumab (TZ)-grafted polyamidoamine dendrimers for selectively targeting HER-2 positive breast cancer cells and delivering docetaxel [57]. *In vitro* experiments demonstrated high antiproliferation activity of targeted dendrimers on HER-2 positive human breast cancer cell line (MDA-MB-435) than on HER-2 negative human breast cell line (MDA-MB-231) when compared with unconjugated dendrimers. The TZ-conjugation of dendrimers also resulted in higher cellular internalization and higher induction of apoptosis against MDA-MB-453 cell lines which indicates that conjugation of trastuzumab on the dendrimer surface helped in the target-specific delivery of docetaxel and reduced systemic toxicity resulting from its off-target effects. The pharmacokinetic parameters of docetaxel were also improved significantly due to conjugation with TZ which was revealed in the *in vivo* studies. Pourianazar *et al.* developed PAMAM dendrimer-coated magnetic nanoparticles and loaded them with CpG-oligodeoxynucleotides. The system had the ability to interact with tumor cells and deliver tumor-killing cargo [58]. CpG-oligodeoxynucleotides function by activating Toll-like receptor 9 (TLR9) by generating cell death cascade. The results showed that the system had high positive charged surfaces which helped in attachment to oligonucleotides electrostatically. The developed PAMAM dendrimer-coated magnetic nanoparticles exhibited higher cellular uptake and cytotoxicity towards both SKBR3 and MDA-MB-231 cell lines compared to uncoated magnetic nanoparticles. In another study, Taghdisi *et al.* developed a dual targeting dendrimer to control the delivery of epirubicin using aptamers of three different kinds (MUC1, AS1411, and ATP aptamers) and evaluated the efficacy in MCF-7 breast cancer cells [59]. The flow cytometry studies revealed that the complex was uptaken by only cancer cells and not by normal cells and this was also confirmed by the MTT assay results. The cytotoxicity of the dendrimer-aptamer complex was less in CHO cells compared to the MCF-7 human breast cancer cells. There was a significant reduction in tumor growth in the *in vivo* studies which demonstrated that this system could treat breast cancer in a pH-sensitive manner. Furthermore, Wang *et al.* designed and developed a pluronic conjugated PAMAM dendrimer using PF-68 for the controlled delivery of DOX [60]. This system was expected to overcome the MDR and reverse it in breast cancer therapy. They have designed a series of PAMAM-Pluronic F68 conjugates. Cytotoxicity studies were carried out in MCF-7/ADR cells by treating with DOX-loaded dendrimer conjugates in tumor spheroids. There was increased antitumor activity of the drug-loaded dendrimer conjugates both *in vitro* and *in vivo*. There was a higher degree of drug accumulation which was due to the caveolae-mediated endocytosis. The system escaped endosomes and lysosomes, and nuclear delivery of DOX was achieved. There was a significant increase in the apoptosis by regulating gene expression and mitochondrial function, overall the PAMAM-PF68 conjugates were significantly effective in overcoming multidrug resistance *in vitro* and *in vivo* and could potentially treat MDR resistant breast cancers.

Summary of different type of dendrimers exploited in the treatment of breast cancer is shown in Table **4**.

Table 4. Dendrimers used in the treatment of breast cancer.

S. No.	Type of Dendrimer	Anti-cancer Therapeutics	*In vitro / In vivo* Model	Outcome	Ref.
1	PAMAM (G4) conjugated with PEG-phospholipid copolymer	DOX and siRNA	MCF-7 and MCF-7/ADR breast cancer cell lines	Localization of cargo, downregulation of p-gp function in MDR cells and higher cytotoxicity thereby MDR reversal.	[52]
2	Tetrabromohydroquinone branched oligoethylene glycol dendrimers	Hydroquinone core of the dendrimers itself	MCF-7 breast cancer cell line	Thermoresponsive dendrimers, D2 dendrimer had the highest cytotoxicity against cancer cells.	[53]

(Table 4) cont.....

S. No.	Type of Dendrimer	Anti-cancer Therapeutics	*In vitro / In vivo* Model	Outcome	Ref.
3	PAMAM-NH$_2$ dendrimer (G3)	Chlorambucil	MCF-7 and MDA-MB-231 breast cancer cell lines	Increased number of apoptotic and necrotic cancer cells, decreased number of viable cells in both cell lines.	[54]
4	PAMAM dendrimer, ethylenediamine core(G4) dendrimer LFC131 conjugate	DOX	BT-549-Luc and T47D breast cancer cell lines	CXCR4 targeted delivery in metastatic cancer cell line, lower migration of cancer cells due to high cytotoxicity.	[55]
5	Polyamidoamine dendrimer (G4)- VEGF-ASODN (antisense oligodeoxynucleotides)	Gene delivery (DNA)	MDA-MB-231 breast cancer cell line, female BALB/cc with MDA-MB-231 breast cancer model	Reduced hemolysis, inhibits tumor vascularization, effective inhibition of breast tumors, and successful gene delivery by protection against restriction enzymes.	[56]
6	PAMAM dendrimer-MAL-PEG-NHS bioconjugate	Trastuzumab	MDA-MB-453 and MDA-M--231 breast cancer cell lines	High antiproliferation in HER2-positive cells, high cell apoptosis and internalization.	[57]
7	3-layer system. Fe$_3$O$_4$ magnetic core, an aminosilane interlayer and a PAMAM dendrimer	CpG-oligodeoxynucleotides	MDA-MB-231 and SKBR3 breast cancer cell lines	Selective drug targeting by application of external magnetic field. Induce cell death in both cell lines.	[58]
8	aptamers-based dendrimers	Epirubicin	MCF-7 breast cancer cell line	Higher cell internalization and cytotoxicity compared to normal cells, targeted delivery and tumor inhibition.	[59]

(Table 4) cont.....

S. No.	Type of Dendrimer	Anti-cancer Therapeutics	*In vitro* / *In vivo* Model	Outcome	Ref.
9	Pluronic conjugated PAMAM dendrimer	DOX	MCF-7/ADR breast cancer cell line, BALB/c mice with MCF-7/ADR tumor spheroid	Higher accumulation due to caveolae mediated endocytosis, higher cytotoxicity, inhibition of tumor spheroids. Bcl-2 MDR gene expression decreased, high biodistribution, significantly overcome MDR, reduced cardiotoxicity.	[60]

POLYMERIC NANOMEDICINE FOR GENE THERAPY IN BREAST CANCER

Gene silencing is rapidly evolving as a personalized approach to breast cancer treatment. The effector molecules—small interfering RNAs (siRNAs), microRNAs (miRNAs) and DNAzyme can be used to silence or "switch off" specific cancer genes. Currently, the main barrier to implementing gene therapies in clinical practice is the lack of an effective delivery system that can protect the gene molecules from nuclease degradation, deliver to them to tumor tissue, and release them into the cytoplasm of the target cancer cells, all without inducing adverse effects [61]. Polymeric nanoparticles offer tremendous promise in addressing most of the challenges associated with siRNA, miRNA and DNAzyme delivery. siRNA has the ability to inhibit or silence different cellular pathways by the destruction of specific mRNA molecules. RNA interference (RNAi) therapies using various siRNA molecules have already been shown to be effective in inhibiting different signalling pathways in cell proliferation and apoptosis. In addition, siRNA has the ability to down-regulate the expression of different multidrug-resistant genes to enhance the accumulation of anticancer drugs at the tumor site [62]. Masjedi *et al.* developed A2AR-specific siRNA loaded PEG-chitosan lactate nanoparticles for interfering with differentiation and function of T cells [63]. Developed siRNA loaded nanoparticles exhibited excellent transfection efficiency in T cells and low toxicity. T cells were treated with A2AR siRNA-loaded NPs demonstrated suppressed expression of A2AR which was associated with increased proliferation, reduced apoptosis, increased the production of inflammatory and reduced secretion of inhibitory cytokines compared to untreated T cells. Moreover, differentiation of conventional T cells purified from tumor-bearing mice to regulatory T cells (Treg) was blocked using A2AR-specific siRNA-loaded NPs. These immune-stimulatory effects were in part through downregulation of protein kinase A/cAMP-response element binding protein (PKA/CREB) axis and upregulation of nuclear factor-κB (NF-κB). In another study, Cui *et al.* developed breast cancer-specific gene 1-small interference RNA (BCSG1-siRNA) plasmid loaded chitosan-silicon dioxide nanoparticles for the treatment of breast cancer [64]. The developed nanoparticles exhibited more than 90% encapsulation efficiency and controlled release profile. The developed siRNA loaded nanoparticles exhibited dose-dependent cytotoxicity towards MCF-7 breast cancer cells.

MicroRNAs (miRNAs) are 22 nucleotide-long, noncoding RNA molecules that act as regulators of gene expression and regulate a range of biological functions, including cell survival, proliferation, apoptosis, tumor growth, and metastasis. miRNAs bind to a complimentary mRNA sequence and result in post-translation repression or degradation and silencing [65]. Wang *et al.* developed HA decorated polyethylenimine-PLGA nanoparticles for targeted co-delivery of DOX and miR-542-3p for TNBC therapy [66]. MiR-542-3p serves as a potent tumor suppressor molecule by targeting tumor suppressor p53 and apoptosis inhibitor survivin. The developed nanoparticle system improved both cellular uptake and cytotoxicity in MDA-MB-231 cells compared to MCF-7 cells, which express lower CD44 levels. Furthermore, intracellular restoration of miR-542-3p further promoted TNBC cell apoptosis *via* activating p53 and inhibiting survivin expression. In another study, Yalcin developed miR29a encapsulated dextran-coated iron oxide nanoparticles for the treatment of breast cancer [67]. The developed nanoparticle system improves the selective delivery of miR29a to the MCF-7 human breast cancer cell line. Moreover, on treatment with miR29a loaded nanoparticle revealed downregulation of anti-apoptotic genes. These results indicate that HA/PEI-PLGA nanoparticles have the potential to co-deliver chemotherapeutic agents and tumor suppressive miRNAs in combinatorial TNBC therapy.

Like other antisense technology, DNAzyme is one of the most promising strategies used to overcome the MDR phenotype and as anticancer agents. One of the new and more efficient ribonucleic acid catalytic methods is DNAzyme that selected through SELEX, which showed higher efficiency, lower toxicity, and faster and more lasting effect compared to others [68]. In this context, Zokaei *et al.* developed mRNA-cleaving DNAzyme loaded chitosan β-cyclodextrin complexes to targets the mRNA of the MDR1 gene in doxorubicin-resistant breast cancer cell line (MCF-7/DR) [69]. Result demonstrated that the developed DNAzyme loaded nanoparticles exhibited 22-fold decrease in DOX resistance after 24 hours of treatment by downregulation of MDR1 mRNAs in MCF-7/DR cells when compared to the control (MCF-7/DR).

CONCLUDING REMARKS

As a rapidly developing interdisciplinary field, cancer nanotechnology brings various perspectives beyond conventional breast cancer treatment that are potentially safer and more efficient. Since the last decades, different biodegradable and biocompatible polymeric nanomedicines have been researched, encapsulated with various chemotherapeutic drugs, and their possible toxicities and different anticancer mechanisms have been investigated. Although, only a few polymeric nanomedicines have managed to enter clinical trials. Therefore, a lot of researches need to be conducted to understand the proper perspective of the polymeric nanomedicines. Polymeric nanomedicines exhibit extraordinary potential for an effective drug delivery system. They have the ability for successful surface decoration, to render imaging and targeting properties, but there are many concerns remains to consider, especially toward clinical trials. Since polymeric nanomedicines are naturally non-immunogenic due to their particle size in nanometer range; therefore, it shows the characteristics of an excellent drug delivery carrier and has ability to reach the target site for therapeutic action. Thus, there is an urgent need to conduct a long period of study to understand the material excretion process and long-term toxicity. In conclusion, the above findings suggested that the polymeric nanomedicines had a great future toward the effective management of breast cancer.

LIST OF ABBREVIATIONS

AURKA Aurora kinase A

CPP Cell-Penetrating Peptide

DOX Doxorubicin

EPR Enhanced Permeability and Retention

ER Estrogen Receptor

HA Hyaluronic Acid

HER2 Human Epidermal Growth Factor Receptor 2

HER-2 Human Epidermal Growth Factor Receptor-2

LHRH Luteinizing Hormone-Releasing Hormone

MDR Multi-Drug Resistance

PAMAM Poly(amidoamine)

PCL Poly(ε-caprolactone)

PDI Polydispersity index

PEG Polyethylene glycol

PLGA Poly (lactide-co-glycolide)

PR	Progesterone Receptor
PTX	Paclitaxel
RES	Reticuloendothelial System
TNBC	Triple Negative Breast Cancer

CONSENT FOR PUBLICATION

Not applicable.

CONFLICT OF INTEREST

The author confirms that this chapter contents have no conflict of interest.

ACKNOWLEDGEMENTS

Declared none.

REFERENCES

[1]   Breast Cancer Facts & Figures 2017-2018. American Cancer Society 2017.

[2]   Waks AG, Winer EP. Breast cancer treatment: A review. JAMA 2019; 321(3): 288-300.
        [http://dx.doi.org/10.1001/jama.2018.19323] [PMID: 30667505]

[3]   Weigelt B, Reis-Filho JS. Histological and molecular types of breast cancer: is there a unifying
        taxonomy? Nat Rev Clin Oncol 2009; 6(12): 718-30.
        [http://dx.doi.org/10.1038/nrclinonc.2009.166] [PMID: 19942925]

[4]   Godone RLN, Leitão GM, Araújo NB, Castelletti CHM, Lima-Filho JL, Martins DBG. Clinical and
        molecular aspects of breast cancer: Targets and therapies. Biomed Pharmacother 2018; 106: 14-34.
        [http://dx.doi.org/10.1016/j.biopha.2018.06.066] [PMID: 29945114]

[5]   Soni K, Rizwanullah M, Kohli K. Development and optimization of sulforaphane-loaded
        nanostructured lipid carriers by the Box-Behnken design for improved oral efficacy against cancer: in
        vitro, ex vivo and in vivo assessments. Artif Cells Nanomed Biotechnol 2018; 46(sup1): 15-31.
        [http://dx.doi.org/10.1080/21691401.2017.1408124] [PMID: 29183147]

[6]   Jain AK, Swarnakar NK, Godugu C, Singh RP, Jain S. The effect of the oral administration of
        polymeric nanoparticles on the efficacy and toxicity of tamoxifen. Biomaterials 2011; 32(2): 503-15.
        [http://dx.doi.org/10.1016/j.biomaterials.2010.09.037] [PMID: 20934747]

[7]   Barkat MA, Rizwanullah M, *et al.* Paclitaxel-loaded nanolipidic carriers with improved oral
        bioavailability and anticancer activity against human liver carcinoma. AAPS PharmSciTech 2019; 20:
        e87.

[8]   Barkat MA, Harshita , Ahmad J, Khan MA, Beg S, Ahmad FJ. Harshita, Ahmad J, Khan MA, Beg S,
        Jalees F. Insights into the targeting potential of thymoquinone for therapeutic intervention against
        triple-negative breast cancer. Curr Drug Targets 2018; 19(1): 70-80.
        [http://dx.doi.org/10.2174/1389450118666170612095959] [PMID: 28606050]

[9]   Foulkes WD, Smith IE, Reis-Filho JS. Triple-negative breast cancer. N Engl J Med 2010; 363(20):
        1938-48.
        [http://dx.doi.org/10.1056/NEJMra1001389] [PMID: 21067385]

[10]   Ahmad J, Akhter S, Greig NH, Kamal MA, Midoux P, Pichon C. Engineered nanoparticles against

MDR in cancer: The state of the art and its prospective. Curr Pharm Des 2016; 22(28): 4360-73.
[http://dx.doi.org/10.2174/1381612822666160617112111] [PMID: 27319945]

[11]   Kutty RV, Wei Leong DT, Feng SS. Nanomedicine for the treatment of triple-negative breast cancer.
       Nanomedicine (Lond) 2014; 9(5): 561-4.
       [http://dx.doi.org/10.2217/nnm.14.19] [PMID: 24827837]

[12]   Rizwanullah M, Amin S, Mir SR, Fakhri KU, Rizvi MMA. Phytochemical based nanomedicines
       against cancer: current status and future prospects. J Drug Target 2018; 26(9): 731-52.
       [http://dx.doi.org/10.1080/1061186X.2017.1408115] [PMID: 29157022]

[13]   Ahmad J, Akhter S, Rizwanullah M, *et al.* Nanotechnology-based inhalation treatments for lung
       cancer: state of the art. Nanotechnol Sci Appl 2015; 8: 55-66.
       [PMID: 26640374]

[14]   Rizwanullah M, Ahmad J, Amin S. Nanostructured lipid carriers: A novel platform for
       chemotherapeutics. Curr Drug Deliv 2016; 13(1): 4-26.
       [http://dx.doi.org/10.2174/1567201812666150817124133] [PMID: 26279117]

[15]   Lee JJ, Saiful Yazan L, Che Abdullah CA. A review on current nanomaterials and their drug conjugate
       for targeted breast cancer treatment. Int J Nanomedicine 2017; 12: 2373-84.
       [http://dx.doi.org/10.2147/IJN.S127329] [PMID: 28392694]

[16]   Dhankhar R, Vyas SP, Jain AK, Arora S, Rath G, Goyal AK. Advances in novel drug delivery
       strategies for breast cancer therapy. Artif Cells Blood Substit Immobil Biotechnol 2010; 38(5): 230-
       49.
       [http://dx.doi.org/10.3109/10731199.2010.494578] [PMID: 20677900]

[17]   Akhter MH, Rizwanullah M, Ahmad J, Ahsan MJ, Mujtaba MA, Amin S. Nanocarriers in advanced
       drug targeting: setting novel paradigm in cancer therapeutics. Artif Cells Nanomed Biotechnol 2018;
       46(5): 873-84.
       [http://dx.doi.org/10.1080/21691401.2017.1366333] [PMID: 28830262]

[18]   Chen J, Li S, Shen Q. Folic acid and cell-penetrating peptide conjugated PLGA-PEG bifunctional
       nanoparticles for vincristine sulfate delivery. Eur J Pharm Sci 2012; 47(2): 430-43.
       [http://dx.doi.org/10.1016/j.ejps.2012.07.002] [PMID: 22796217]

[19]   Choi JS, Jang WS, Park JS. Comparison of adsorption and conjugation of Herceptin on poly(lactic-c-
       -glycolic acid) nanoparticles - Effect on cell internalization in breast cancer cells. Mater Sci Eng C
       2018; 92: 496-507.
       [http://dx.doi.org/10.1016/j.msec.2018.06.059] [PMID: 30184775]

[20]   Cerqueira BBS, Lasham A, Shelling AN, Al-Kassas R. Development of biodegradable PLGA
       nanoparticles surface engineered with hyaluronic acid for targeted delivery of paclitaxel to triple
       negative breast cancer cells. Mater Sci Eng C 2017; 76: 593-600.
       [http://dx.doi.org/10.1016/j.msec.2017.03.121] [PMID: 28482569]

[21]   Talaei F, Azizi E, Dinarvand R, Atyabi F. Thiolated chitosan nanoparticles as a delivery system for
       antisense therapy: evaluation against EGFR in T47D breast cancer cells. Int J Nanomedicine 2011; 6:
       1963-75.
       [PMID: 21976973]

[22]   Dong S, Guo Y, Duan Y, *et al.* Co-delivery of paclitaxel and gemcitabine by methoxy poly(ethylene
       glycol)-poly(lactide-coglycolide)-polypeptide nanoparticles for effective breast cancer therapy.
       Anticancer Drugs 2018; 29(7): 637-45.
       [http://dx.doi.org/10.1097/CAD.0000000000000631] [PMID: 29846247]

[23]   Eatemadi A, Daraee H, Aiyelabegan HT, Negahdari B, Rajeian B, Zarghami N. Synthesis and
       Characterization of Chrysin-loaded PCL-PEG-PCL nanoparticle and its effect on breast cancer cell
       line. Biomed Pharmacother 2016; 84: 1915-22.
       [http://dx.doi.org/10.1016/j.biopha.2016.10.095] [PMID: 27847208]

[24]   Anari E, Akbarzadeh A, Zarghami N. Chrysin-loaded PLGA-PEG nanoparticles designed for enhanced effect on the breast cancer cell line. Artif Cells Nanomed Biotechnol 2016; 44(6): 1410-6. [PMID: 26148177]

[25]   Mishra B, Padaliya R, Patel RR. Exemestane encapsulated vitamin E-TPGS-polymeric nanoparticles: preparation, optimization, characterization, and *in vitro* cytotoxicity assessment. Artif Cells Nanomed Biotechnol 2017; 45(3): 522-34. [http://dx.doi.org/10.3109/21691401.2016.1163714] [PMID: 27017970]

[26]   Ghanghoria R, Tekade RK, Mishra AK, Chuttani K, Jain NK. Luteinizing hormone-releasing hormone peptide tethered nanoparticulate system for enhanced antitumoral efficacy of paclitaxel. Nanomedicine (Lond) 2016; 11(7): 797-816. [http://dx.doi.org/10.2217/nnm.16.19] [PMID: 26980704]

[27]   Saxena V, Naguib Y, Hussain MD. Folate receptor targeted 17-allylamino--7-demethoxygeldanamycin (17-AAG) loaded polymeric nanoparticles for breast cancer. Colloids Surf B Biointerfaces 2012; 94: 274-80. [http://dx.doi.org/10.1016/j.colsurfb.2012.02.001] [PMID: 22377218]

[28]   Hashad RA, Ishak RAH, Geneidi AS, Mansour S. Surface functionalization of methotrexate-loaded chitosan nanoparticles with hyaluronic acid/human serum albumin: Comparative characterization and *in vitro* cytotoxicity. Int J Pharm 2017; 522(1-2): 128-36. [http://dx.doi.org/10.1016/j.ijpharm.2017.03.008] [PMID: 28279742]

[29]   de Oliveira Pedro R, Hoffmann S, Pereira S, Goycoolea FM, Schmitt CC, Neumann MG. Self-assembled amphiphilic chitosan nanoparticles for quercetin delivery to breast cancer cells. Eur J Pharm Biopharm 2018; 131: 203-10. [http://dx.doi.org/10.1016/j.ejpb.2018.08.009] [PMID: 30145220]

[30]   Ercan A, Çelebier M, Varan G, *et al.* Global omics strategies to investigate the effect of cyclodextrin nanoparticles on MCF-7 breast cancer cells. Eur J Pharm Sci 2018; 123: 377-86. [http://dx.doi.org/10.1016/j.ejps.2018.07.060] [PMID: 30076952]

[31]   Greish K, Mathur A, Al Zahrani R, *et al.* Synthetic cannabinoids nano-micelles for the management of triple negative breast cancer. J Control Release 2018; 291: 184-95. [http://dx.doi.org/10.1016/j.jconrel.2018.10.030] [PMID: 30367922]

[32]   Logie J, Ganesh AN, Aman AM, Al-Awar RS, Shoichet MS. Preclinical evaluation of taxane-binding peptide-modified polymeric micelles loaded with docetaxel in an orthotopic breast cancer mouse model. Biomaterials 2017; 123: 39-47. [http://dx.doi.org/10.1016/j.biomaterials.2017.01.026] [PMID: 28161682]

[33]   Lu J, Zhao W, Huang Y, *et al.* Targeted delivery of Doxorubicin by folic acid-decorated dual functional nanocarrier. Mol Pharm 2014; 11(11): 4164-78. [http://dx.doi.org/10.1021/mp500389v] [PMID: 25265550]

[34]   Mahdaviani P, Bahadorikhalili S, Navaei-Nigjeh M, *et al.* Peptide functionalized poly ethylene glycol-poly caprolactone nanomicelles for specific cabazitaxel delivery to metastatic breast cancer cells. Mater Sci Eng C 2017; 80: 301-12. [http://dx.doi.org/10.1016/j.msec.2017.05.126] [PMID: 28866169]

[35]   Kheiri Manjili H, Ghasemi P, Malvandi H, Mousavi MS, Attari E, Danafar H. Pharmacokinetics and *in vivo* delivery of curcumin by copolymeric mPEG-PCL micelles. Eur J Pharm Biopharm 2017; 116: 17-30. [http://dx.doi.org/10.1016/j.ejpb.2016.10.003] [PMID: 27756682]

[36]   Nosrati H, Barzegari P, Danafar H, Kheiri Manjili H. Biotin-functionalized copolymeric PEG-PCL micelles for *in vivo* tumour-targeted delivery of artemisinin. Artif Cells Nanomed Biotechnol 2019; 47(1): 104-14. [http://dx.doi.org/10.1080/21691401.2018.1543199] [PMID: 30663422]

[37]   Guo Y, He W, Yang S, Zhao D, Li Z, Luan Y. Co-delivery of docetaxel and verapamil by reduction-sensitive PEG-PLGA-SS-DTX conjugate micelles to reverse the multi-drug resistance of breast cancer. Colloids Surf B Biointerfaces 2017; 151: 119-27.
[http://dx.doi.org/10.1016/j.colsurfb.2016.12.012] [PMID: 27988472]

[38]   Saxena V, Hussain MD. Poloxamer 407/TPGS mixed micelles for delivery of gambogic acid to breast and multidrug-resistant cancer. Int J Nanomedicine 2012; 7: 713-21.
[PMID: 22359450]

[39]   Qiu JF, Gao X, Wang BL, *et al.* Preparation and characterization of monomethoxy poly(ethylene glycol)-poly(ε-caprolactone) micelles for the solubilization and in vivo delivery of luteolin. Int J Nanomedicine 2013; 8: 3061-9.
[PMID: 23990719]

[40]   Guzzarlamudi S, Singh PK, Pawar VK, *et al.* Synergistic chemotherapeutic activity of curcumin bearing methoxypolyethylene glycol-g-linoleic acid based micelles on breast cancer cells. J Nanosci Nanotechnol 2016; 16(4): 4180-90.
[http://dx.doi.org/10.1166/jnn.2016.11699] [PMID: 27451784]

[41]   Thakur CK, Thotakura N, Kumar R, *et al.* Chitosan-modified PLGA polymeric nanocarriers with better delivery potential for tamoxifen. Int J Biol Macromol 2016; 93(Pt A): 381-9.
[http://dx.doi.org/10.1016/j.ijbiomac.2016.08.080] [PMID: 27586640]

[42]   Zhang R, Su S, Hu K, *et al.* Smart micelle@polydopamine core-shell nanoparticles for highly effective chemo-photothermal combination therapy. Nanoscale 2015; 7(46): 19722-31.
[http://dx.doi.org/10.1039/C5NR04828A] [PMID: 26556382]

[43]   Wang Y, Chen L, Tan L, *et al.* PEG-PCL based micelle hydrogels as oral docetaxel delivery systems for breast cancer therapy. Biomaterials 2014; 35(25): 6972-85.
[http://dx.doi.org/10.1016/j.biomaterials.2014.04.099] [PMID: 24836952]

[44]   Song C, Sun H, Zhang L, Ma G, He Y. Paclitaxel-loaded polymeric micelles based on poly(ε-caprolactone)-poly(ethylene glycol)-poly(ε-caprolactone) triblock copolymers: *in vitro* and *in vivo* evaluation. Nanomedicine (Lond) 2011; 8: 925-34.

[45]   Hadinoto K, Sundaresan A, Cheow WS. Lipid-polymer hybrid nanoparticles as a new generation therapeutic delivery platform: a review. Eur J Pharm Biopharm 2013; 85(3 Pt A): 427-43.
[http://dx.doi.org/10.1016/j.ejpb.2013.07.002] [PMID: 23872180]

[46]   Du M, Ouyang Y, Meng F, *et al.* Polymer-lipid hybrid nanoparticles: A novel drug delivery system for enhancing the activity of Psoralen against breast cancer. Int J Pharm 2019; 561: 274-82.
[http://dx.doi.org/10.1016/j.ijpharm.2019.03.006] [PMID: 30851393]

[47]   Tian F, Dahmani FZ, Qiao J, *et al.* A targeted nanoplatform co-delivering chemotherapeutic and antiangiogenic drugs as a tool to reverse multidrug resistance in breast cancer. Acta Biomater 2018; 75: 398-412.
[http://dx.doi.org/10.1016/j.actbio.2018.05.050] [PMID: 29874597]

[48]   Monirinasab H, Asadi H, Rostamizadeh K, Esmaeilzadeh A, Khodaei M, Fathi M. Novel lipid-polymer hybrid nanoparticles for siRNA delivery and IGF-1R gene silencing in breast cancer cells. J Drug Deliv Sci Technol 2018; 48: 96-105.
[http://dx.doi.org/10.1016/j.jddst.2018.08.025]

[49]   Yang Z, Luo X, Zhang X, Liu J, Jiang Q. Targeted delivery of 10-hydroxycamptothecin to human breast cancers by cyclic RGD-modified lipid-polymer hybrid nanoparticles. Biomed Mater 2013; 8(2): 025012.
[http://dx.doi.org/10.1088/1748-6041/8/2/025012] [PMID: 23507576]

[50]   Zhang RX, Cai P, Zhang T, *et al.* Polymer-lipid hybrid nanoparticles synchronize pharmacokinetics of co-encapsulated doxorubicin-mitomycin C and enable their spatiotemporal co-delivery and local bioavailability in breast tumor. Nanomedicine (Lond) 2016; 12(5): 1279-90.

[http://dx.doi.org/10.1016/j.nano.2015.12.383] [PMID: 26772427]

[51]   Zhao P, Wang H, Yu M, *et al.* Paclitaxel loaded folic acid targeted nanoparticles of mixed lipid-shell and polymer-core: *in vitro* and *in vivo* evaluation. Eur J Pharm Biopharm 2012; 81(2): 248-56.
[http://dx.doi.org/10.1016/j.ejpb.2012.03.004] [PMID: 22446630]

[52]   Pan J, Mendes LP, Yao M, *et al.* Polyamidoamine dendrimers-based nanomedicine for combination therapy with siRNA and chemotherapeutics to overcome multidrug resistance. Eur J Pharm Biopharm 2019; 136: 18-28.
[http://dx.doi.org/10.1016/j.ejpb.2019.01.006] [PMID: 30633973]

[53]   Abdel-Rahman MA, Al-Abd AM. Thermoresponsive dendrimers based on oligoethylene glycols: design, synthesis and cytotoxic activity against MCF-7 breast cancer cells. Eur J Med Chem 2013; 69: 848-54.
[http://dx.doi.org/10.1016/j.ejmech.2013.09.019] [PMID: 24121308]

[54]   Bielawski K, Bielawska A, Muszyńska A, Popławska B, Czarnomysy R. Cytotoxic activity of G3 PAMAM-NH$_2$ dendrimer-chlorambucil conjugate in human breast cancer cells. Environ Toxicol Pharmacol 2011; 32(3): 364-72.
[http://dx.doi.org/10.1016/j.etap.2011.08.002] [PMID: 22004955]

[55]   Chittasupho C, Anuchapreeda S, Sarisuta N. CXCR4 targeted dendrimer for anti-cancer drug delivery and breast cancer cell migration inhibition. Eur J Pharm Biopharm 2017; 119: 310-21.
[http://dx.doi.org/10.1016/j.ejpb.2017.07.003] [PMID: 28694161]

[56]   Wang P, Zhao XH, Wang ZY, Meng M, Li X, Ning Q. Generation 4 polyamidoamine dendrimers is a novel candidate of nano-carrier for gene delivery agents in breast cancer treatment. Cancer Lett 2010; 298(1): 34-49.
[http://dx.doi.org/10.1016/j.canlet.2010.06.001] [PMID: 20594639]

[57]   Kulhari H, Pooja D, Shrivastava S, *et al.* Trastuzumab-grafted PAMAM dendrimers for the selective delivery of anticancer drugs to HER2-positive breast cancer. Sci Rep 2016; 6: 23179.
[http://dx.doi.org/10.1038/srep23179] [PMID: 27052896]

[58]   Taghavi Pourianazar N, Gunduz U. CpG oligodeoxynucleotide-loaded PAMAM dendrimer-coated magnetic nanoparticles promote apoptosis in breast cancer cells. Biomed Pharmacother 2016; 78: 81-91.
[http://dx.doi.org/10.1016/j.biopha.2016.01.002] [PMID: 26898428]

[59]   Taghdisi SM, Danesh NM, Ramezani M, *et al.* Double targeting and aptamer-assisted controlled release delivery of epirubicin to cancer cells by aptamers-based dendrimer *in vitro* and *in vivo*. Eur J Pharm Biopharm 2016; 102: 152-8.
[http://dx.doi.org/10.1016/j.ejpb.2016.03.013] [PMID: 26987703]

[60]   Wang M, Li Y, HuangFu M, *et al.* Pluronic-attached polyamidoamine dendrimer conjugates overcome drug resistance in breast cancer. Nanomedicine (Lond) 2016; 11(22): 2917-34.
[http://dx.doi.org/10.2217/nnm-2016-0252] [PMID: 27780403]

[61]   Ahmadzada T, Reid G, McKenzie DR. Fundamentals of siRNA and miRNA therapeutics and a review of targeted nanoparticle delivery systems in breast cancer. Biophys Rev 2018; 10(1): 69-86.
[http://dx.doi.org/10.1007/s12551-017-0392-1] [PMID: 29327101]

[62]   Mahmoodi Chalbatani G, Dana H, Gharagouzloo E, *et al.* Small interfering RNAs (siRNAs) in cancer therapy: a nano-based approach. Int J Nanomedicine 2019; 14: 3111-28.
[http://dx.doi.org/10.2147/IJN.S200253] [PMID: 31118626]

[63]   Masjedi A, Hassannia H, Atyabi F, *et al.* Downregulation of A2AR by siRNA loaded PEG-chitosa--lactate nanoparticles restores the T cell mediated anti-tumor responses through blockage of PKA/CREB signaling pathway. Int J Biol Macromol 2019; 133: 436-45.
[http://dx.doi.org/10.1016/j.ijbiomac.2019.03.223] [PMID: 30936011]

[64]   Cui L, Zheng R, Liu W, *et al.* Preparation of chitosan-silicon dioxide/BCSG1-siRNA nanoparticles to

enhance therapeutic efficacy in breast cancer cells. Mol Med Rep 2018; 17(1): 436-41.
[PMID: 29115613]

[65]   Ganju A, Khan S, Hafeez BB, *et al.* miRNA nanotherapeutics for cancer. Drug Discov Today 2017;
22(2): 424-32.
[http://dx.doi.org/10.1016/j.drudis.2016.10.014] [PMID: 27815139]

[66]   Wang S, Zhang J, Wang Y, Chen M. Hyaluronic acid-coated PEI-PLGA nanoparticles mediated co-
delivery of doxorubicin and miR-542-3p for triple negative breast cancer therapy. Nanomedicine
(Lond) 2016; 12(2): 411-20.
[http://dx.doi.org/10.1016/j.nano.2015.09.014] [PMID: 26711968]

[67]   Yalcin S. Dextran-coated iron oxide nanoparticle for delivery of miR-29a to breast cancer cell line.
Pharm Dev Technol 2019; 24(8): 1032-7.
[http://dx.doi.org/10.1080/10837450.2019.1623252] [PMID: 31159615]

[68]   Fokina AA, Stetsenko DA, François JC. DNA enzymes as potential therapeutics: towards clinical
application of 10-23 DNAzymes. Expert Opin Biol Ther 2015; 15(5): 689-711.
[http://dx.doi.org/10.1517/14712598.2015.1025048] [PMID: 25772532]

[69]   Zokaei E, Badoei-Dalfrad A, Ansari M, Karami Z, Eslaminejad T, Nematollahi-Mahani SN.
Therapeutic potential of DNAzyme loaded on chitosan/cyclodextrin nanoparticle to recovery of
chemosensitivity in the MCF-7 cell line. Appl Biochem Biotechnol 2019; 187(3): 708-23.
[http://dx.doi.org/10.1007/s12010-018-2836-x] [PMID: 30039475]

CHAPTER 3

Treatment of Lung Cancer in the New Era

Girisha Maheshwari, Bhanu Pratap Chauhan, Shweta Dang and **Reema Gabrani**[*]

Jaypee Institute of Information Technology, A-10, Sector 62, Noida, Uttar Pradesh, India

Abstract: The most frequent cancer related deaths have been associated with lung cancer. The subtypes, Non-Small Cell Lung Cancer (NSCLC) and Small Cell Lung Cancers (SCLC), respond to chemical drugs and radiotherapy. NSCLC (60%) express membrane epidermal growth factor receptor (EGFR). The cell signalling pathway induced by EGFR has been attributed as a key reason for lung cancer progression. There are many FDA approved drugs available for the treatment which primarily includes EGFR tyrosine kinase inhibitors (TKIs) such as erlotinib and gefitinib, or EGFR neutralizing antibody, necitumumab. However, the reports suggest that EGFR can undergo further mutation in tyrosine kinase domain which makes the cells resistant to the ongoing treatment. Alternate signalling pathways may get activated accompanied by epithelial mesenchymal transition and imbalanced microRNAs that contribute towards resistance. Epigenetic changes in lung cancer also offer dynamic targets for cancer therapy. The agents targeting epigenetic changes can be combined with chemotherapy or other-directed therapy so that effective dose and hence toxicity is reduced with enhanced efficacy. Micro-RNAs are the largest class of the gene regulators that regulate the cancer genes. Inhibiting or replacing the cancer-causing miRNAs can be potential targets for cancer treatment. Researchers have also worked on immunotherapy drugs like nivolumab, pembrolizumab and atezolizumab, which reverse the inhibitory mechanism of the immune response. New findings from recent trails provide an optimistic perspective on the progress towards the better treatment of lung cancer.

Keywords: EGFR, Epigenetic, Immunotherapy, miRNA, PD-1/PDL-1, T790M mutation.

INTRODUCTION

Lung cancer or lung carcinoma is defined as the uncontrolled proliferation of normal lung cells due to the genetic damage and it has the capacity to invade the neighboring tissues and metastasize the various cells of the body. Lung Cells sometimes behave abnormally and do not grow; these changes may lead to nonca-

[*] **Corresponding author Reema Gabrani:** Jaypee Institute of Information Technology, A-10, Sector 62, Noida, Uttar Pradesh, India; Tel: +91-120-2594211; E-mail: reema.gabrani@jiit.ac.in

Atta-ur-Rahman and M. Iqbal Choudhary (Eds.)

ncerous tumors like hamartoma and papilloma. On the other hand, some changes that develops into cancerous behaviour with the ability to metastasize to different organs [1]. Today, in the 20th century, lung cancer is reported for the most deaths at the worldwide level and ranked high in both incidence and mortality. Lung cancer is subdivided into two forms: Non-Small Cell Lung Cancer (NSCLC) and Small-Cell Lung Cancer (SCLC) where NSCLC are considered as the most prevalent form. Lung Cancer was considered a rare disease till the beginning of the 19th century whereas, thereafter increased incidents of lung cancer cases have been linked to rising in cigarette consumption worldwide [2]. Cigarette or tobacco contains benzo[a] pyrene, nicotine-derived nitrosamine ketone, 1, 3-butadiene and radioisotope of polonium-210, polonium among which at least 73 known carcinogens are identified and are the main reasons for lung cancer. Apart from smoking, the inheritance of gene polymorphism, radiations, asbestos and air pollution have also been found to be the major reasons for lung cancer [3].

The genetic DNA damage and epigenetic changes affect the cellular normal function, proliferation, repair, and apoptosis [4]. Molecular alterations in phosphoinositide 3-Kinase (PI3K)/Protein kinase B also known as AKT/mammalian target of rapamycin (mTor) pathways have been linked to lung cancer. Certain biomarkers like ProGRP (pro-gastrin-releasing peptide), CEACAM (carcinoembryonic antigen), EPCAM (epithelial cell adhesion molecule) and CYFRA 21-1 (cytokeratins) have been reported for their use in the diagnosis of lung cancer. Successful chemotherapy regimens were developed in 1970 after that new chemotherapy drugs for NSCLC include paclitaxel, docetaxel, vinorelbine, and gemcitabine [5]. Patients that were found with genomic aberrations are benefitted with the molecular targeted therapies. Some of the current therapies have been listed in Fig. (**1**). Epidermal Growth Factor Receptor (EGFR) overexpression has been predominantly linked to NSCLC lung cancer and has been related to poor survival and increased metastasis. Gefitinib and Erlotinib are the first generation reversible inhibitors that can completely block the adenosine triphosphate (ATP) binding site of EGFR and also inhibit the activity of tyrosine kinase. Unfortunately, there are many types of cancer that acquire resistance mutations and stop responding to the drugs. Although new drugs have been developed which are sensitive to the mutated versions of the EGFR, there is still a need to explore more compounds and drugs which could be effective against lung cancer [6].

SMALL MOLECULE-BASED INHIBITORS

The discovery and optimization of small molecule inhibitors for the treatment of human diseases have been the major focus of the pharmaceutical industry for more than a century. Small-molecule kinase inhibitors are being intensively pursued as new anticancer therapeutics. Broadly, there are three categories of inhibitors that are mentioned in Table **1**. Currently, there are some of the known kinase inhibitors that target the ATP binding site with the kinase activation loop in the active (Type 1) or inactive (Type 2) conformations [19].

Table 1. Recent FDA approved drugs used for the treatment of Non-small cell lung cancer [7].

S.No	Name of Inhibitor	Year of Approval	Mechanism of Action	References
First Generation Inhibitors				
1.	Crizotinib (Xalkori)	March 11, 2016	An anti-cancer drug for Anaplastic lymphoma kinase (ALK) or ROS1 (c-ros oncogene-1) positive metastatic NSCLC.	[8]
2.	Erlotinib Hydrochloride (Tarceva)	May 14, 2013	It competes for the ATP binding site of EGFR and further inhibits phosphorylation of tyrosine kinase.	[9]
3.	Gefitinib (Iressa)	May 5, 2003	It blocks the ATP binding site which in turn inhibits the tyrosine kinase activity of EGFR.	[10]
Second Generation Inhibitors				
4.	Dacomitinib (Vizimpro)	September 27, 2018	Dacomitinib is used for the first-line treatment for metastatic NSCLC with EGFR exon 19 deletion or exon 21 L858R substitution mutations.	[11]
5.	Afatinib Dimaleate (Gilotrif)	January 12, 2018	Afatinib is used to treat metastatic NSCLC where tumors have non-resistant EGFR mutations.	[12]
6.	Alectinib (Alecensa)	November 6, 2017	Alectinib is used as an oral drug to block the activity of ALK to treat NSCLC.	[13]
7.	Ceritinib (Zykadia)	May 26, 2017	Ceritinib is used for the treatment of ALK-positive metastatic NSCLC.	[14]
8.	Brigatinib (Alunbrig)	April. 28, 2017	Inhibitor for metastatic NSCLC having alteration in ALK gene.	[15]
Third Generation Inhibitors				
9.	Lorlatinib (Lorbrena)	November 2, 2018	ALK-positive metastatic NSCLC resistant to crizotinib/ alectinib or ceritinib.	[16]
10.	Osimertinib Mesylate (Tagrisso)	March 30, 2017	Irreversible inhibitor, targets metastatic EGFR T790M mutation harboring NSCLC.	[17]
11.	Olmutinib (Olita)	May 2016	Irreversible TKI binds tyrosine kinase domain of mutant EGFR.	[18]

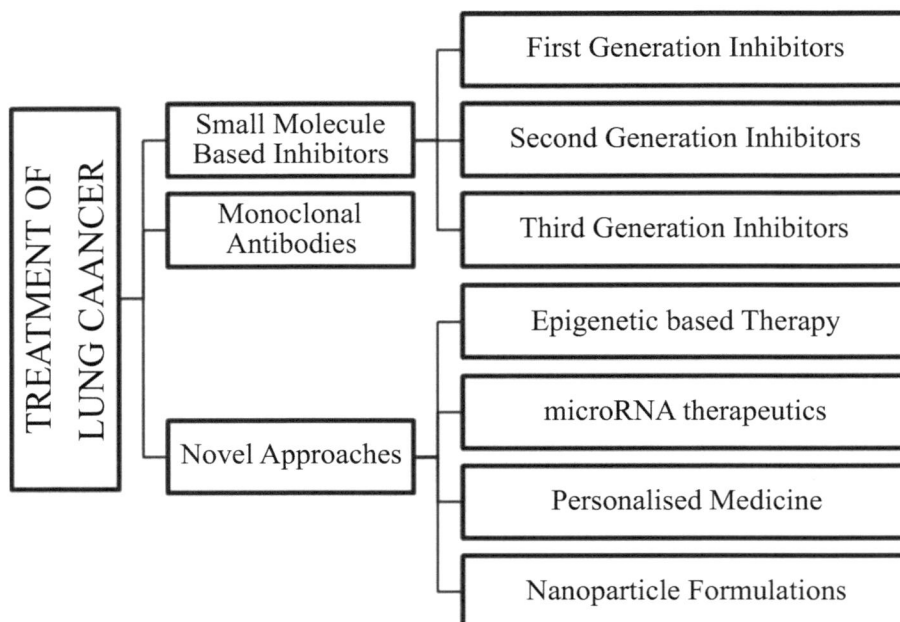

Fig. (1). Approaches to the treatment of lung cancer.

First Generation Inhibitors

Discovery of activating mutations in EGFR as a predictive biomarker for first-generation EGFR TKIs has been initiated as an era of precision oncology for the treatment of advanced EGFR-mutant NSCLC [20]. When the ligand binds to the receptor, its dimerization leads to the activation (phosphorylation) and EGFR activates downstream PI-3-K, and mitogen-activated protein kinases pathways which can regulate key cellular processes which leads to proliferation and apoptosis. EGFR can also induce angiogenesis and metastasis and thus support tumor growth. Therefore, targeting EGFR has been strongly pursued so that new or improved version of molecular inhibitors could be scrutinized. The finding of new molecules that can target the tyrosine kinase of EGFR unlocks a new way of managing advanced NSCLC. The EGFR specific TKIs, gefitinib [20] and erlotinib are molecularly targeted drugs that are used for the treatment of NSCLC [21, 22].

Gefitinib is an orally given TKI that binds to EGFR and is a well-tolerated treatment for advanced NSCLC [10]. Gefitinib was the first agent designed to get the U.S. Food and Drug Administration (FDA) approval with a known molecular target and is also acclaimed for the treatment of lung cancer. Gefitinib is a low-molecular-weight synthetic anilinoquinazoline that has a specific mechanism to inhibit the phosphorylation as well as TK activity by competitively binding to the intracellular ATP-binding site of EGFR. Erlotinib hydrochloride is an EGFR inhibitor that inhibits tyrosine phosphorylation in EGFR; as a result, there is no signal cascade [9, 21, 22].

Second Generation Inhibitors

Second-generation EGFR TKIs have been developed to overcome the resistance which develops while targeting first-generation inhibitors. Resistance to EGFR TKIs in NSCLCs is activated by two key mechanisms namely secondary mutation Thr790Met in EGFR and c-mesenchymal-epithelial transition factor (c-Met) amplification. Several therapeutic approaches are being researched which can overcome TKI resistance. Second-generation EGFR TKIs have been invented to overcome the resistance by inhibiting human EGFR 2 (HER2) and EGFR by binding in an irreversible fashion to the kinase domain [23]. Examples of inhibitors are dacomitinib (Vizimpro) and afatinib (Gilotrif) [23]. Dacomitinib can irreversibly inhibit EGFR, HER2 and HER4 as compared to gefitinib/erlotinib and it shows a higher kinase inhibition and is also able to target EGFR-T790M and HER2-mutated cell lines [11]. Afatinib which is another second-generation EGFR TKI is also used orally and binds to EGFR, HER2, and HER4 in an irreversible manner and can target cells harbouring EGFR mutations including T790M mutation [12, 24].

Third Generation Inhibitors

Osimertinib (Tagrisso), a third-generation EGFR-TKI, has been approved by the FDA in March, 2017 for the treatment of EGFR-mutated NSCLCs [25]. The main feature of osimertinib is that it is mutant selective and it mainly targets EGFR mutant cells as compared to EGFR wild type cells [26]. Osimertinib targets EGFR mutations that covers T790M and have shown resistance to first/ second generation TKIs [27]. The lung cancer patients who have EGFR T790M mutation as tested by the Cobas EGFR mutation test is approved to be treated by osimertinib. This compound has also received an additional FDA approval as first-line therapy for suppressing the mutation in EGFR (exon 21 L858R) and deletion in its exon 19 and thus contributes to patient's progression free survival [17]. The third-generation compounds at various stages of development are mavelertinib (PF-0647775), olmutinib (Olita), an orally active EGFR inhibitor used in the treatment of T790M mutation positive NSCLC [16]. Nazartinib (EGF816), a third-generation EGFR TKI that selectively targets activating (L858R, ex19del) and resistance (T790M) mutants seems promising in clinical trials [27 - 29].

MONOCLONAL ANTIBODIES

Monoclonal antibodies are highly specific antibodies that can bind to their epitopes and facilitate to target the tumor-specific or associated antigens. The monoclonal antibodies which are accepted to treat the NSCLC (adenocarcinoma) are summarized in Table **2**. There are proteins located on the cancer cells which act as the binding site for monoclonal antibodies. This binding of monoclonal antibodies to the cancer cells helps to mount the immune response and destroy tumor cells. The PD-1 and cytotoxic T-lymphocyte–associated antigen 4 (CTLA-4) pathways are the immune checkpoints that are critical for the ability of the immune system to control cancer cell growth. There are a number of cancer cells that use PD-1 and CTLA-4 pathways to escape the immune system as they down regulate T cells function. Specific antibodies or immune checkpoint inhibitors block these pathways and help the immune system to respond towards the cancer cells. Once the immune system recognises these cancer cells, it can slow down or stop the cancer cell growth. Immunotherapy is mainly divided into two parts that are passive and active immunotherapy. Any immunologically active agent that does not rely on host machinery and is made *in vitro* is called passive immunotherapy. The passive immunotherapy includes the monoclonal antibody that binds to the specific ligands present on tumor cells, for example, trastuzumab or herceptin which targets HER2 and avastin which recognizes vascular endothelial growth factor (VEGF) [37]. Active immunotherapy targets the host's immune system to stimulate the specific immune response to a disease. The primary objective of active immunotherapy is the induction of antigen-specific T-cell. The immune system has several checkpoints that slow down or stop an immune system attack when the healthy cells are exposed. The drugs which are being explored for the treatment of lung cancer to boost immune response are called checkpoint inhibitors [38, 39].

Table 2. **Monoclonal antibody-based inhibitors for lung cancer. Brand names are mentioned in brackets.**

Molecule	Targeted Site	Mechanism Of Action	References
Bevacizumab (Avastin Mvasi)	Vascular endothelial growth factor (VEGF)	Specifically, binds to VEGF and prevents interaction with its receptor. FDA approved for metastatic NSCLC in combination with carboplatin and paclitaxel	[30]
Nivolumab (Opdivo)	Programmed death receptor-1 (PD-1)	Induces the programmed tumor cell death by binding to the Programmed cell death receptor-1 (PD-1).	[31]
Pembrolizumab (Keytruda)	PD-1 molecule	Blocks PD-1 on T cells and prevents their exhaustion; first-line treatment for stage III nonsquamous NSCLC	[32]

(Table 2) cont.....

Molecule	Targeted Site	Mechanism Of Action	References
Atezolizumab (Tecentriq)	Programmed death ligand-1 (PD-L1) molecule	Binds PD-L1 on tumor cells; The first-line treatment for metastatic NSCLC having no EGFR/ ALK mutations.	[33]
Ramucirumab (Cyramza)	Vascular endothelial growth factor receptor 2 (VEGFR2)	Ramucirumab is an anti-angiogenic agent that targets and binds VEGFR-2 for NSCLC.	[34]
Necitumumab (Portrazza)	EGFR	Necitumumab is directed against the binding domain of EGFR, approved for the treatment of NSCLC in combination with cisplatin-gemcitabine.	[35]
Durvalumab (Imfinzi)	Programmed death-ligand 1 (PD-L1)	Binds to PD-L1 on tumor cells, removes the block on activation of T cells	[36]

Aberrant EGFR expression is being directly linked to lung cancer and necitumumab is FDA approved to bind and block the receptor dimerization and activation. Necitumumab is the first line treatment for squamous NSCLC which has metastatized. During clinical trials necitumumab in combination with gemcitabine and cisplatin exhibited significant improvement [35]. VEGF promotes neovascularisation and is also responsible for improved endothelial cell proliferation and their survival which leads to tumor growth and metastasis. VEGF is the activator of angiogenesis that stimulates the migration and proliferation of endothelial cells in existing vessels to generate and stabilize new blood vessels. VEGF is released in hypoxic conditions as an effect of the hypoxia-inducible factor (HIF-1α) and causes re-modulation and inflammation of bronchi cell. Cell re-modulation and inflammation lead to the development of various lung disorders like pulmonary hypertension, chronic obstructive pulmonary disease, asthma, fibrosis, and lung cancer. Various natural and synthetic drugs are available for reducing the overexpression of VEGF and FGF-2 which can be helpful in treating lung disorders. One such example is bevacizumab which is a humanized monoclonal antibody and is also an anti-VEGF drug that binds to VEGF to abolish the chance of activation of vascular endothelial growth factor receptor (VEGFR), thereby exerting an anti-angiogenic effect [40]. Bevacizumab is approved to be used for metastatic NSCLC along with carboplatin, paclitaxel and atezolizumab.

Another important marker which has been identified is programmed cell death ligand (PDL-1)/ Programmed cell death protein 1 (PD-1) checkpoint.

The PD-1 is expressed on T-cells, B-cells and natural killer T-cells [40]. PD-1 presence on leukocytes and its interaction with PDL-1 contributes to tolerance to self tissue especially in peripheral region. PDL-1 is expressed on tumor cells and it suppresses the immune system and inhibits the activation of T cells. The FDA has approved the use of atezolizumab, nivolumab [31] and pembrolizumab as second-line therapy for advanced NSCLC with disease progression on or after platinum-containing chemotherapy. Atezolizumab is approved as first line treatment along with other drugs for metastatic NSCLC harbouring no mutations in EGFR and ALK. It is also indicated as first line treatment for ES-SCLC patients in association with carboplatin and etoposide [41].

Another monoclonal antibody that inhibits PD-1 molecule is nivolumab and it further causes the programmed death of tumor cells [31]. Monoclonal antibody blocks the interaction between PD-1 and PDL-1 to prevent T cell exhaustion [37, 38].

Currently, research is focussed on extending the uses of already approved monoclonal antibodies or combining with other drugs. Nimotuzumab is a humanized IgG1 isotype monoclonal antibody which constrains the binding of EGFR to cancer cells [42]. Nimotuzumab is approved for squamous cell carcinoma in the head and neck in many countries. The studies suggest that nimotuzumab can be combined with chemotherapy and also cisplatin for the improved efficacy against NSCLC [43].

Lung cancer can metastasize into the bone and complicates the treatment. Nuclear factor-kappa B signaling plays an important role in bone resorption by osteoclasts. Denosumab is a human monoclonal antibody and it binds to the nuclear factor-kappa B ligand (RANKL) and reduces tumor growth in bone. According to the recent studies, it has been observed that the denosumab could increase the survival rate in the patients with metastatic lung cancer [44, 45].

NOVEL APPROACHES

Epigenetic Therapies

Epigenetic therapy undertakes novel, inventive treatment options to target and help in the treatment of lung cancer. The two recognised therapies are DNA methyltransferase inhibitors (DNMTi) and the agents which modify histones [46]. DNA methylation of the promoter region of tumor suppressor gene in human lung cancer can inhibit its expression. The epigenetic modifications in cooperation with the histone tail changes can also alter the chromatin remodelling [47]. Azacitidine and 5-aza-2′-deoxycytidine (decitabine) are two types of clinically approved DNMTi that are generally noted as the flagships of epigenetic therapy. Rather than being cytotoxic as normal chemotherapeutics, epigenetic therapies promote apoptosis or differentiation by silencing or the activation of genes. Lung cancer patients may get benefit from the epigenetically positive drugs in combination with chemotherapy. It is also suitable for high-risk NSCLC patients who otherwise do not respond well to chemotherapy. High-risk NSCLC patients with less relapse-free survival seem to be susceptible to drugs targeting relevant epigenetic alterations like DNA methylation of HIST1H4F, PCDHGB6, NPBWR1, ALX1, and HOXA. Epigenetic changes have been identified as putative cancer biomarkers for early detection, disease monitoring, prognosis, and risk assessment [47].

MicroRNA

MicroRNAs (miRNAs) are long non-coding RNAs that either degrade mRNA or translationally repress of mRNA by negatively regulating the expression of tumor suppressor genes as explained in Fig. (**2**) [48]. miRNAs are small molecules that play a key role in the regulation of basic cellular processes, including differentiation, proliferation, and apoptosis by controlled gene expression at the post-transcriptional level [49]. It is also confirmed that miRNAs play a part in epithelial-mesenchymal transition, which is an important feature of metastasis during lung cancer development [50]. They are a valuable tool not only in treatment but also diagnosis of lung cancer.

Tumor Supressor MicroRNAs in Lung Cancer

The patients diagnosed with lung cancer were found to have decreased levels of Let-7 as compared to the normal person. Let-7 in normal cells downregulates the expression of RAS protein, a key messenger for the MAPK pathway. Thus, overexpression of RAS protein in lung cancer has been linked to a decrease in the number of transcripts of let-7 [50, 51].

The studies have shown that when miR-126 is overexpressed in the lung cancer cell lines, it reduces the Crk protein which results in fixation and diminished migration. Crk protein arbitrates many intracellular signal pathways, which are accountable for cell growth, fixation, differentiation, and motility. The overexpression of miR-126 also reduces the expression of VEGF. The miRNA-145 suppresses c-myc, a key transcription factor during cell-cell cycle and also inhibits cell growth and overexpression by blocking G1/S transition in A549 and H23 cells. The miR-34 family consists of miR-34a, -34b and -34c and shows anti-tumorigenic nature. miR-34 family induces apoptosis and cell cycle arrest in cancer cells by directly regulating p53 [52].

Oncogenic MicroRNA in Lung Cancer

The miRNAs whose expression is increased in tumors may be called as oncogenes. These oncogene miRNAs are also called as "oncomirs", that generally promote tumor development by negatively inhibiting tumor suppressor genes and/or genes that control cell differentiation or apoptosis [53]. The miRNA-17-92 cluster reduces the γ-H2AX foci, marker for DNA double-stranded breaks, which in turn counterbalances the DNA damage. Inhibition of miR-17-5p and miR20a, part of cluster miR-17-92, by antisense oligonucleotides results in apoptosis of lung cancer cells. Overexpression of miR-21 upregulates Ras-MAPK pathway and inhibits apoptosis. It directly targets 3'-UTR of human muts homolog2 which in turn affects the cell proliferation and cell cycle in cell lines of NSCLC [54]. Knockdown of miR-31-5p increases hMLH1 protein expression and induces apoptosis. These findings reveal the oncogenic function of mir-31. The miR-221 and mir-222 contribute to cellular migration by increasing signalling of MMPs and AKT pathway. They can directly target the metalloproteinase 3 tumor suppressors and PTEN which induces TRAIL resistance and also enhances cellular migration [55].

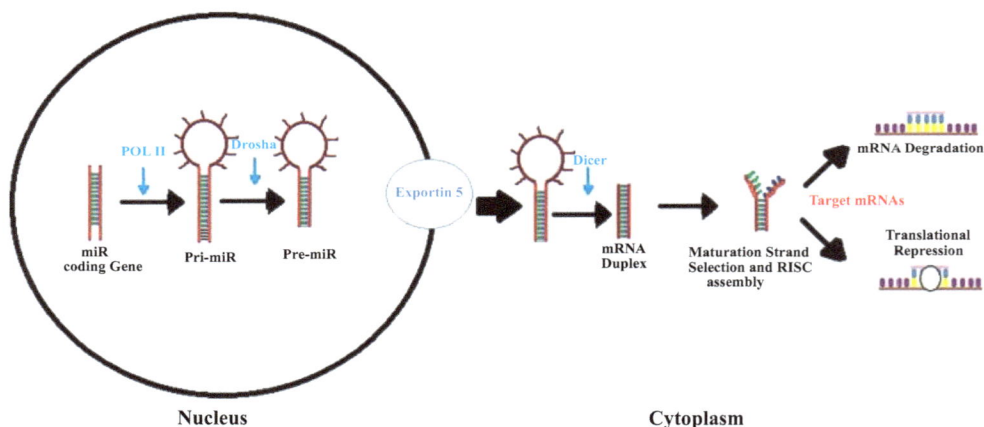

Fig. (2). Processing of miRNA and RNA induced silencing complex (RISC) assembly.

NANOPARTICLE FORMULATIONS

Nanoencapsulated drugs can assist in diagnosis as well as therapeutics of cancer. The types of nanosystems being studied for lung cancer are polymeric micelles, dendrimers, liposomes and lipid nanoparticles [56, 57]. Paclitaxel loaded nanoparticles (Abraxane) have been indicated for NSCLC by US-FDA along with carboplatin. Abraxane is less toxic and promotes cell death in G2 and M stages of cell cycle by stabilizing microtubules.

Inhibitor (BMS-202) targeting PD-1/ PDL-1 interaction has been encapsulated for enhanced penetration and longer retention at tumor site to boost the immune response [58]. Apart from drugs, nanoencapsualted siRNA is being investigated for its efficacy and effective delivery as viable treatment option [59].

PERSONALIZED MEDICINE

Cancer is a multi-step process where every patient has different molecular signature and hence heterogeneity is observed even for same type of cancer. This leads to complexity at genome, tumor stage and histological manifestation [60]. This underlines the importance of personalized medicine. With the advent of next generation sequencing and reduction in cost analysis, detection of specific mutation is feasible. Personalized medicine can be achieved by targeting the specific sites/mutations associated with lung cancer. First line of treatment for aberrant expression of EGFR in lung cancer is TKIs gefitinb and erlotinib [61]. Accumulation of specific mutations like L858R and T790M in EGFR led to the development of next generation TKIs dacomitinib and osimertinib, respectively. This emphasizes the fact that tumor which develops resistance to drugs needs to be genetically mapped and specific therapeutic agents need to be developed to target these altered proteins/miRNAs. Apart from EGFR, specific mutations in lung cancer have been identified in ALK, K-RAS, MET and ROS proteins. Monoclonal antibodies have also been established to target the specific interaction between ligand and receptor [62]. Atezolizumab, nivolumab and pembrolizumab target PD-1/PDL-1 interaction and enhance the T cell response towards tumor cells. Increased reports of resistance to single drug treatment have changed the focus to the development of admixture or synergistic combination of drugs. Knowledge of specific mutations or genome signature will help in redefining the current treatment and paving way for personalized medicine [63].

CONCLUSION

The most frequent deaths have been related to lung cancer. Lung cancer is generally of two types that is NSCLC and SCLC. There are many FDA approved drugs that are available for the treatment which mainly include EGFR TKIs, erlotinib and gefitinib or EGFR neutralizing antibody necitumumab. Gefitinib was the first-generation inhibitor designed to bind known molecular target and received the FDA approval for the treatment of NSCLC. The second-generation EGFR TKIs have been developed so that it could address the resistance to inhibitors used in first line treatment for lung cancer. The examples of the second-generation EGFR TKIs are dacomitinib, and afatinib. Osimertinib, a third-generation TKI, has been approved for the treatment of resistant/mutant EGFR in NSCLC. Monoclonal antibodies are being extensively researched and are getting approvals in recent years for the treatment of lung cancer. Monoclonal antibodies were highly specific to their epitopes can target the tumor specific or associated antigens. The monoclonal antibodies which are approved for the treatment of NSCLC include nivolumab, pembrolizumab, and bevacizumab. The novel approaches include the epigenetic therapies which cover DNMT inhibitors and the agents which modify histones. Another novel approach is by manipulating the levels of miRNAs. They are the non-coding RNAs that either degrade mRNA or do translational repression of mRNA by negatively regulating the expression of the cancer- related genes by sequence selection targeting of mRNA. Nano encapsulated drugs are being explored to address delivery issues, improve bioavailability and reduce toxicity and abraxane is indicated for metastatic NSCLC. Genome mapping and identification of signature mutations/changes associated with cancer is paving the way towards personalized medicine. Focus is shifting towards the use of combination therapy for wide and specific targeting and simultaneously minimizing toxicity and resistance to existing drugs.

CONSENT FOR PUBLICATION

Not applicable.

CONFLICT OF INTEREST

The author confirms that this chapter contents have no conflict of interest.

ACKNOWLEDGEMENTS

Declared none.

REFERENCES

[1]   Alberg AJ, Brock MV, Ford JG, Samet JM, Spivack SD. Epidemiology of lung cancer: Diagnosis and management of lung cancer, 3rd ed: American College of Chest Physicians evidence-based clinical practice guidelines. Chest 2013; 143(5) (Suppl.): e1S-e29S.
        [http://dx.doi.org/10.1378/chest.12-2345] [PMID: 23649439]

[2]   Siegel R, Naishadham D, Jemal A. Cancer statistics, 2013. CA Cancer J Clin 2013; 63(1): 11-30.
        [http://dx.doi.org/10.3322/caac.21166] [PMID: 23335087]

[3]   Shigematsu H, Lin L, Takahashi T, *et al.* Clinical and biological features associated with epidermal growth factor receptor gene mutations in lung cancers. J Natl Cancer Inst 2005; 97(5): 339-46.
        [http://dx.doi.org/10.1093/jnci/dji055] [PMID: 15741570]

[4]   Nasim F, Sabath BF, Eapen GA. Lung Cancer. Med Clin North Am 2019; 103(3): 463-73.
        [http://dx.doi.org/10.1016/j.mcna.2018.12.006] [PMID: 30955514]

[5]   Virnig BA, Baxter NN, Habermann EB, Feldman RD, Bradley CJ. A matter of race: early-versus late-stage cancer diagnosis. Health Aff (Millwood) 2009; 28(1): 160-8.
        [http://dx.doi.org/10.1377/hlthaff.28.1.160] [PMID: 19124866]

[6]   Kelly RJ, Shepherd FA, Krivoshik A, Jie F, Horn L. A phase III, randomized, open-label study of ASP8273 versus erlotinib or gefitinib in patients with advanced stage IIIB/IV non-small-cell lung cancer. Ann Oncol 2019; 30(7): 1127-33.
        [http://dx.doi.org/10.1093/annonc/mdz128] [PMID: 31070709]

[7]   US Food and Drug Administration. Hematology/oncology (cancer) approvals & safety notifications, 2016. Available from FDA. http://www.fda.gov/Drugs/InformationOnDrugs/ApprovedDrugs/ucm 279174

[8]   Shaw AT, Kim DW, Nakagawa K, *et al.* Crizotinib versus chemotherapy in advanced ALK-positive lung cancer. N Engl J Med 2013; 368(25): 2385-94.
[http://dx.doi.org/10.1056/NEJMoa1214886] [PMID: 23724913]

[9]   D'Arcangelo M, Cappuzzo F. Erlotinib in the first-line treatment of non-small-cell lung cancer. Expert Rev Anticancer Ther 2013; 13(5): 523-33.
[http://dx.doi.org/10.1586/era.13.23] [PMID: 23617344]

[10]   Cohen MH, Williams GA, Sridhara R, *et al.* United States Food and Drug Administration drug approval summary: gefitinib (ZD1839; Iressa) tablets. Clin Cancer Res 2004; 10(4): 1212-8.
[http://dx.doi.org/10.1158/1078-0432.CCR-03-0564] [PMID: 14977817]

[11]   Ou SH, Soo RA. Dacomitinib in lung cancer: a "lost generation" EGFR tyrosine-kinase inhibitor from a bygone era? Drug Des Devel Ther 2015; 9(1177): 5641-53.
[http://dx.doi.org/10.2147/DDDT.S52787] [PMID: 26508839]

[12]   Yang JC-H, Shih J-Y, Su W-C, *et al.* Afatinib for patients with lung adenocarcinoma and epidermal growth factor receptor mutations (LUX-Lung 2): a phase 2 trial. Lancet Oncol 2012; 13(5): 539-48.
[http://dx.doi.org/10.1016/S1470-2045(12)70086-4] [PMID: 22452895]

[13]   Avrillon V, Pérol M. Alectinib for treatment of ALK-positive non-small-cell lung cancer. Future Oncol 2017; 13(4): 321-35.
[http://dx.doi.org/10.2217/fon-2016-0386] [PMID: 27780368]

[14]   Shaw AT, Kim DW, Mehra R, *et al.* Ceritinib in ALK-rearranged non-small-cell lung cancer. N Engl J Med 2014; 370(13): 1189-97.
[http://dx.doi.org/10.1056/NEJMoa1311107] [PMID: 24670165]

[15]   Hegedüs C, Truta-Feles K, Antalffy G, *et al.* Interaction of the EGFR inhibitors gefitinib, vandetanib, pelitinib and neratinib with the ABCG2 multidrug transporter: implications for the emergence and reversal of cancer drug resistance. Biochem Pharmacol 2012; 84(3) 2 60-7
[http://dx.doi.org/10.1016/j.bcp.2012.04.010]

[16]   US Food and Drug Administration. FDA approves lorlatinib for second-or third-line treatment of ALK-positive metastatic NSCLC 2019. https://www.fda.gov/drugs/fda-approves-lorlatinib-second-or-third-line-treatment-alk-positive-metastatic-nsclc

[17]   Santarpia M, Liguori A, Karachaliou N, *et al.* Osimertinib in the treatment of non-small-cell lung cancer: design, development and place in therapy. Lung Cancer (Auckl) 2017; 8: 109-25.
[http://dx.doi.org/10.2147/LCTT.S119644] [PMID: 28860885]

[18]   Kim ES. Olmutinib: first global approval. Drugs 2016; 76(11): 1153-7.
[http://dx.doi.org/10.1007/s40265-016-0606-z] [PMID: 27357069]

[19]   Roskoski R Jr. Small molecule inhibitors targeting the EGFR/ErbB family of protein-tyrosine kinases in human cancers. Pharmacol Res 2019; 139: 395-411.
[http://dx.doi.org/10.1016/j.phrs.2018.11.014] [PMID: 30500458]

[20]   Maemondo M, Inoue A, Kobayashi K, *et al.* Gefitinib or chemotherapy for non-small-cell lung cancer with mutated EGFR. N Engl J Med 2010; 362(25): 2380-8.
[http://dx.doi.org/10.1056/NEJMoa0909530] [PMID: 20573926]

[21]   Shepherd FA, Rodrigues Pereira J, Ciuleanu T, *et al.* National Cancer Institute of Canada Clinical Trials Group. Erlotinib in previously treated non-small-cell lung cancer. N Engl J Med 2005; 353(2): 123-32.
[http://dx.doi.org/10.1056/NEJMoa050753] [PMID: 16014882]

[22]   Karachaliou N, Codony-Servat J, Bracht JWP, *et al.* Characterising acquired resistance to erlotinib in

non-small cell lung cancer patients. Expert Rev Respir Med 2019; 13(10): 1019-28.
[http://dx.doi.org/10.1080/17476348.2019.1656068] [PMID: 31411906]

[23] Shu D, Xu Y, Chen W. Knockdown of lncRNA BLACAT1 reverses the resistance of afatinib to non-small cell lung cancer *via* modulating STAT3 signaling. J Drug Target 2020; 28(3): 300-6.

[24] Taniguchi Y, Yamamoto M, Ikushima H, *et al.* Successful Treatment of Afatinib-Refractory Non-Small Cell Lung Cancer with Uncommon Complex EGFR Mutations Using Pembrolizumab: A Case Report. Case Rep Oncol 2019; 12(2): 564-7.
[http://dx.doi.org/10.1159/000501848] [PMID: 31427953]

[25] Zhang YC, Zhou Q, Wu YL. Clinical management of third-generation EGFR inhibitor-resistant patients with advanced non-small cell lung cancer: Current status and future perspectives. Cancer Lett 2019; 459: 240-7.
[http://dx.doi.org/10.1016/j.canlet.2019.05.044] [PMID: 31201840]

[26] Bollinger MK, Agnew AS, Mascara GP. Osimertinib: A third-generation tyrosine kinase inhibitor for treatment of epidermal growth factor receptor-mutated non-small cell lung cancer with the acquired Thr790Met mutation. J Oncol Pharm Pract 2018; 24(5): 379-88.
[http://dx.doi.org/10.1177/1078155217712401] [PMID: 28565936]

[27] Jiang T, Su C, Ren S, *et al.* written on behalf of the AME Lung Cancer Collaborative Group. A consensus on the role of osimertinib in non-small cell lung cancer from the AME Lung Cancer Collaborative Group. J Thorac Dis 2018; 10(7): 3909-21.
[http://dx.doi.org/10.21037/jtd.2018.07.61] [PMID: 30174832]

[28] Soria JC, Ohe Y, Vansteenkiste J, *et al.* Osimertinib in untreated EGFR-mutated advanced non–small-cell lung cancer N Engl J Med 2018 2018; 378(2) 113-25.

[29] Murtuza A, Bulbul A, Shen JP, *et al.* Novel third-generation EGFR tyrosine kinase inhibitors and strategies to overcome therapeutic resistance in lung cancer. Cancer Res 2019; 79(4): 689-98.
[http://dx.doi.org/10.1158/0008-5472.CAN-18-1281] [PMID: 30718357]

[30] Assoun S, Brosseau S, Steinmetz C, Gounant V, Zalcman G. Bevacizumab in advanced lung cancer: state of the art. Future Oncol 2017; 13(28): 2515-35.
[http://dx.doi.org/10.2217/fon-2017-0302] [PMID: 28812378]

[31] Kazandjian D, Suzman DL, Blumenthal G, *et al.* FDA approval summary: nivolumab for the treatment of metastatic non-small cell lung cancer with progression on or after platinum-based chemotherapy. Oncologist 2016; 21(5): 634-42.
[http://dx.doi.org/10.1634/theoncologist.2015-0507] [PMID: 26984449]

[32] Qin Q, Li B. Pembrolizumab for the treatment of nonsmall cell lung cancer: Current status and future directions. J Cancer Res Ther 2019; 15(4): 743-50.
[http://dx.doi.org/10.4103/jcrt.JCRT_903_18] [PMID: 31436226]

[33] Vansteenkiste J, Wauters E, Park K, Rittmeyer A, Sandler A, Spira A. Prospects and progress of atezolizumab in non-small cell lung cancer. Expert Opin Biol Ther 2017; 17(6): 781-9.
[http://dx.doi.org/10.1080/14712598.2017.1309389] [PMID: 28335643]

[34] Arrieta O, Zatarain-Barrón ZL, Cardona AF, Carmona A, Lopez-Mejia M. Ramucirumab in the treatment of non-small cell lung cancer. Expert Opin Drug Saf 2017; 16(5): 637-44.
[http://dx.doi.org/10.1080/14740338.2017.1313226] [PMID: 28395526]

[35] Brinkmeyer JK, Moore DC. Necitumumab for the treatment of squamous cell non-small cell lung cancer. J Oncol Pharm Pract 2018; 24(1): 37-41.
[http://dx.doi.org/10.1177/1078155216682365] [PMID: 27913776]

[36] US Food and drug administration. 2017. Available from:. https://dailymed.nlm.nih.gov/dailymed/fda/fdaDrugXsl.cfm?setid=8baba4ea-2855-42fa-9bd9-5a7548d4cec3

[37] Laddha AP, Kulkarni YA. VEGF and FGF-2: Promising targets for the treatment of respiratory disorders. Respir Med 2019; 156(1532): 33-46.

[http://dx.doi.org/10.1016/j.rmed.2019.08.003] [PMID: 31421589]

[38]   Xu P, Li H. Application of bevacizumab in non-small cell lung cancer. Zhongguo Fei Ai Za Zhi 2017; 20(4): 272-7.
[PMID: 28442017]

[39]   Silva AP, Coelho PV, Anazetti M, Simioni PU. Targeted therapies for the treatment of non-small-cell lung cancer: Monoclonal antibodies and biological inhibitors. Hum Vaccin Immunother 2017; 13(4): 843-53.
[http://dx.doi.org/10.1080/21645515.2016.1249551] [PMID: 27831000]

[40]   Frezzetti D, Gallo M, Maiello MR, *et al.* VEGF as a potential target in lung cancer. Expert Opin Ther Targets 2017; 21(10): 959-66.
[http://dx.doi.org/10.1080/14728222.2017.1371137] [PMID: 28831824]

[41]   Tsoukalas N, Kiakou M, Tsapakidis K, *et al.* PD-1 and PD-L1 as immunotherapy targets and biomarkers in non-small cell lung cancer. J BUON 2019; 24(3): 883-8.
[PMID: 31424637]

[42]   Si X, Wu S, Wang H, *et al.* Nimotuzumab combined with chemotherapy as first-line treatment for advanced lung squamous cell carcinoma. Thorac Cancer 2018; 9(8): 1056-61.
[http://dx.doi.org/10.1111/1759-7714.12789] [PMID: 29920955]

[43]   Yang Y, Zhou W, Wu J, *et al.* Antitumor activity of nimotuzumab in combination with cisplatin in lung cancer cell line A549 *in vitro*. Oncol Lett 2018; 15(4): 5280-4.
[http://dx.doi.org/10.3892/ol.2018.7923] [PMID: 29552167]

[44]   De Castro J, García R, Garrido P, *et al.* Therapeutic potential of denosumab in patients with lung cancer: Beyond prevention of skeletal complications. Clin Lung Cancer 2015; 16(6): 431-46.
[http://dx.doi.org/10.1016/j.cllc.2015.06.004] [PMID: 26264596]

[45]   Chen Y, Li J, Chen S, *et al.* Nab-paclitaxel in combination with cisplatin versus docetaxel plus cisplatin as first-line therapy in non-small cell lung cancer. Sci Rep 2017; 7(1): 10760.
[http://dx.doi.org/10.1038/s41598-017-11404-9] [PMID: 28883517]

[46]   Shinjo K, Kondo Y. Clinical implications of epigenetic alterations in human thoracic malignancies: epigenetic alterations in lung cancer. Methods Mol Biol 2012; 863: 221-39.
[http://dx.doi.org/10.1007/978-1-61779-612-8_13] [PMID: 22359296]

[47]   Brait M, Sidransky D. Cancer epigenetics: above and beyond. Toxicol Mech Methods 2011; 21(4): 275-88.
[http://dx.doi.org/10.3109/15376516.2011.562671] [PMID: 21495866]

[48]   Lopez-Serra P, Esteller M. DNA methylation-associated silencing of tumor-suppressor microRNAs in cancer. Oncogene 2012; 31(13): 1609-22.
[http://dx.doi.org/10.1038/onc.2011.354] [PMID: 21860412]

[49]   Florczuk M, Szpechcinski A, Chorostowska-Wynimko J. miRNAs as biomarkers and therapeutic targets in non-small cell lung cancer: Current perspectives. Target Oncol 2017; 12(2): 179-200.
[http://dx.doi.org/10.1007/s11523-017-0478-5] [PMID: 28243959]

[50]   Lin PY, Yu SL, Yang PC. MicroRNA in lung cancer. Br J Cancer 2010; 103(8): 1144-8.
[http://dx.doi.org/10.1038/sj.bjc.6605901] [PMID: 20859290]

[51]   Akao Y, Nakagawa Y, Naoe T. let-7 microRNA functions as a potential growth suppressor in human colon cancer cells. Biol Pharm Bull 2006; 29(5): 903-6.
[http://dx.doi.org/10.1248/bpb.29.903] [PMID: 16651716]

[52]   Zhang B, Pan X, Cobb GP, Anderson TA. microRNAs as oncogenes and tumor suppressors. Dev Biol 2007; 302(1): 1-12.
[http://dx.doi.org/10.1016/j.ydbio.2006.08.028] [PMID: 16989803]

[53]   Esquela-Kerscher A, Slack FJ. Oncomirs - microRNAs with a role in cancer. Nat Rev Cancer 2006;

6(4): 259-69.
[http://dx.doi.org/10.1038/nrc1840] [PMID: 16557279]

[54]   Wang V, Wu W. MicroRNA-based therapeutics for cancer. BioDrugs 2009; 23(1): 15-23.
[http://dx.doi.org/10.2165/00063030-200923010-00002] [PMID: 19344188]

[55]   Hussain S. Nanomedicine for Treatment of Lung Cancer. Adv Exp Med Biol 2016; 890: 137-47.
[http://dx.doi.org/10.1007/978-3-319-24932-2_8] [PMID: 26703803]

[56]   Lee HY, Mohammed KA, Nasreen N. Nanoparticle-based targeted gene therapy for lung cancer. Am J
Cancer Res 2016; 6(5): 1118-34.
[PMID: 27294004]

[57]   Wang XS, Zhang L, Li X, *et al.* Nanoformulated paclitaxel and AZD9291 synergistically eradicate
non-small-cell lung cancers *in vivo.* Nanomedicine (Lond) 2018; 13(10): 1107-20.
[http://dx.doi.org/10.2217/nnm-2017-0355] [PMID: 29874151]

[58]   Zhang R, Zhu Z, Lv H, *et al.* Immune checkpoint blockade mediated by a small-molecule
nanoinhibitor targeting the PD-1/PD-L1 pathway synergizes with photodynamic therapy to elicit
antitumor immunity and antimetastatic effects on breast cancer. Small 2019; 15(49): e1903881.
[http://dx.doi.org/10.1002/smll.201903881] [PMID: 31702880]

[59]   Itani R, Al Faraj A. siRNA conjugated nanoparticles-a next generation strategy to treat lung cancer. Int
J Mol Sci 2019; 20(23): E6088.
[http://dx.doi.org/10.3390/ijms20236088] [PMID: 31816851]

[60]   Mascaux C, Tomasini P, Greillier L, Barlesi F. Personalised medicine for nonsmall cell lung cancer.
Eur Respir Rev 2017; 26(146): 170066.
[http://dx.doi.org/10.1183/16000617.0066-2017] [PMID: 29141962]

[61]   Jiang W, Cai G, Hu PC, Wang Y. Personalized medicine in non-small cell lung cancer: a review from
a pharmacogenomics perspective. Acta Pharm Sin B 2018; 8(4): 530-8.
[http://dx.doi.org/10.1016/j.apsb.2018.04.005] [PMID: 30109178]

[62]   Hensing T, Chawla A, Batra R, Salgia R. A personalized treatment for lung cancer: molecular
pathways, targeted therapies, and genomic characterization. Adv Exp Med Biol 2014; 799: 85-117.
[http://dx.doi.org/10.1007/978-1-4614-8778-4_5] [PMID: 24292963]

[63]   Mok TS. Personalized medicine in lung cancer: what we need to know. Nat Rev Clin Oncol 2011;
8(11): 661-8.
[http://dx.doi.org/10.1038/nrclinonc.2011.126] [PMID: 21862980]

CHAPTER 4

Oral Administration of Cancer Chemotherapeutics Exploiting Self-Nanoemulsifying Drug Delivery System: Recent Progress and Application

Javed Ahmad[1], Farooq Ali Khan[2], Mohammad Zaki Ahmad[1], Showkat Rasool Mir[3], Noor Alam[4] and Saima Amin[5,*]

[1] *Department of Pharmaceutics, College of Pharmacy, Najran University, Najran, KSA*

[2] *Sri Indu Institute of Pharmacy, Hyderabad, India*

[3] *Phytopharmaceutical Research Laboratory, School of Pharmaceutical Education and Research, Jamia Hamdard, New Delhi, India*

[4] *Post-Graduate Department of Botany, Purnea University, Bihar, India*

[5] *Department of Pharmaceutics, School of Pharmaceutical Education and Research, Jamia Hamdard, New Delhi, India*

Abstract: The delivery of cancer chemotherapeutics has shifted dramatically in the last two decades from parenteral to oral administration. Improved patient compliance, drug tolerability, ease of administration, and potential effectiveness for oral therapy relative to intravenous administration have appeared as the main reasons to use cancer chemotherapeutics through the oral route of administration. However, most of the cancer chemotherapeutics show very poor oral absorption due to the drug's physicochemical characteristics, stability, and biological barrier (multidrug efflux proteins: P-glycoproteins) present in the GI tract. With advanced research in homolipids and heterolipids as excipients, lipid-based formulations were exploited to enhance the oral efficacy of poorly absorbable cancer chemotherapeutics in recent years. Self-nanoemulsifying drug delivery system (SNEDDS) is the highly developed strategy of emulsion dependent drug delivery systems and relies on the GI fluids for the formation of nanoemulsion inside the *in vivo* system. The advancement in the field of biocompatible lipid and their derivatives in addition to finding on pharmaceutical excipients such as oil, surfactants, co-surfactants having P-gp modulating potential further extend the interest in SNEDDS for delivery of cancer chemotherapeutics through oral administration. This chapter provides a comprehensive discussion about contemporary advancement in the application of SNEDDS for oral delivery of cancer chemotherapeutics.

* **Corresponding author Saima Amin:** Department of Pharmaceutics, School of Pharmaceutical Education and Research, Jamia Hamdard, New Delhi, India; E-mail:samin@jamiahamdard.ac.in; daneshyarsaima@yahoo.com

Atta-ur-Rahman and M. Iqbal Choudhary (Eds.)

Keywords: Cancer Chemotherapeutics, Nanoemulsion, Oral Absorption, P-Glycoproteins, SNEDDS.

INTRODUCTION

Cancer is a disease that occurs after numerous mutagenesis steps, permitting cancerous cells to develop uncontrollably [1]. Cancer is a leading cause of global mortalities. The cancer burden rises to 18.1 million new cases and 9.6 million cancer deaths in 2018. The diagnoses estimated for different cancers are: cancer of lung (2.1 million), breast (2.1 million), colorectal (1.8 million), prostate (1.3 million), and stomach (1.0 million) [2]. Breast cancer is the most common form of cancer in women globally and is rising mainly in developing countries where most of the cases are diagnosed in later stages [3]. The recent data from the World Health Organization suggests a 45% increase in the deaths caused due to cancer by 2030, of which 70% would be in developing countries like India [2]. Owing to these figures, there is a growing concern to treat this deadly disease. Presently, the technologies have made huge development but accurate therapy is still a challenge. Existing cancer treatments can be widely classified into two groups: cytotoxic therapies and molecular targeted drug delivery [4, 5]. Except for a few cancer types, where the treatment involves hormonal therapy or immunotherapy, cytotoxic agents remain the major form of chemotherapy for cancer [6]. Cytotoxic agents are a diverse class of compounds that are used in cancer therapy as they are toxic to cells that grow and divide quickly. Due to the fast growth and proliferation of cancerous cells, they are favorably killed by these agents. The preferred routes of administering these cytotoxic agents are through intravenous bolus or infusion, usually in the form of a drug solution. They have been used for a long time and the development of several multi-drug treatment regimens improved their clinical success. However, there is still the case of treatment failure [7, 8]. There is often an enormous and erratic protein binding of cytotoxic agents with body tissue and serum protein when given through traditional mode, only a small portion of the cytotoxic agents reach the tumor site [9]. This generally reduces the therapeutic efficacy and increases the systemic toxicity of the drug. Cytotoxic agents are supposed to kill only the cancer cells; however, they also end up killing noncancerous cells such as the ones which quickly divide, *e.g.* bone marrow cells. There is a regular occurrence of normal tissue toxicities even when the dose of anticancer agents remains standard. The significant challenge to effective cancer treatment is the poor drug specificity in terms of biodistribution and also at the cellular levels. The patients' quality of life and the overall life expectancy relates directly to the targeting ability of cytotoxic agents. Systemic administration through intravenous bolus or infusion sometimes leads to side effects which can be at times so intense, that the patient has to discontinue the therapy, even before the drug could kill cancer cells [10]. There is an evolution of new anticancer agents and also the development of new methods to effectively administer old drugs.

ANTICANCER ORAL THERAPY

In oncology, medicines as chemotherapy are mostly delivered intravenously contrasting the majority of biomedical disciplines [11, 12]. There has been a dramatic shift in the administration of chemotherapeutic agents, they are now been given orally differing from the traditional parenteral route. However, the administration of cancer chemotherapeutics has shifted remarkably in the past 15 years from parenteral to oral administration [13, 14]. During recent times, the therapeutic trends have been observed by a continuous growth in the availability of oral cytotoxic drugs with >20 oral anti-cancer drugs presently approved for application in the United States and Europe [15 - 17]. It has mostly been the preference of patients to choose oral therapy relative to intravenous administration simply because of ease of administration and home-based therapy. It is also required that the toxicities associated with oral therapy should not be higher than intravenous therapy and the efficacy should be the same. Improved compliance, tolerance, ease of administration, and potential efficacy for oral therapy relative to intravenous administration have appeared as the major cause to use cancer chemotherapeutics through oral delivery. Compliance is vital for oral therapy because it decides the dose-intensity of the therapy and eventually efficacy and toxicity of the therapy. A lot of surveys indicate that maximum patients favor oral therapy to intravenous therapy [18 - 20]. Liu and group found that 89% of patients favor oral therapy rather than intravenous. It is primarily for the convenience of a home-based therapy (57% of patients), thereby escaping the insertion of a venous catheter (55% of patients) [18]. Other reasons were the negative earlier experiences with intravenous administration and a lesser access rate to the oncology service. The oral administration of cytotoxic agents provides longer drug exposure when compared to intermittent intravenous infusion. The drug exposure is dependent on exponential factors which are concentration and time. A drug with shorter $t_{1/2}$ achieves better exposure time when given as a nonstop infusion. The exposure time has profound effects on drug toxicities and efficacy. An added advantage of oral chemotherapy is the decrease in the utilization of various resources for inpatient and ambulatory care services. There is also an improved quality of life with oral chemotherapy. Despite their numerous advantages for convenience and patient compliance, there are however potential challenges with the oral use of chemotherapeutic agents, which clinicians are desired to be aware of and take necessary steps to circumvent them or mitigate them [21 - 23]. Lastly, keeping in mind the rising prices of anticancer therapy, oral therapy of cytotoxic agents is appealing as it avoids the requirement of hospitalization, doctors, paramedical staff, and infusion tools. However, most of the chemotherapeutics (for instance paclitaxel, doxorubicin, cisplatin, *etc.*) show very poor oral absorption due to the drug's physicochemical characteristics, stability and biological barrier (P-glycoproteins: multidrug efflux pumps) present in the GI tract [24 - 26]. Before the systemic absorption, the drug has to go through various biological events including dissolution in GI fluid, passing through the GI epithelial or transmembrane transport in different pH conditions, pre-systemic metabolism, and efflux *via* multidrug efflux proteins [27, 28]. Considering the above challenges that lead to low drug availability, significant efforts have been made in this area for the success of anticancer oral therapy.

BIOPHARMACEUTICAL BARRIERS IN ORAL CHEMOTHERAPY

The factors which determine the oral absorption of any therapeutics rely on its solubility and stability in the gastrointestinal fluid as well as permeability through intestinal epithelium, and the pre-systemic metabolism [29, 30]. Various barriers that obstruct the success of anticancer oral therapy mainly include physiological barriers and biochemical barriers [31]. Physicochemical characteristics of the cancer chemotherapeutics are well investigated and found to be significantly influencing its oral absorption. The log P and pKa of anticancer therapeutics which indicate the lipophilicity and extent of drug ionization may directly influence its oral absorption [32]. The majority of anticancer drugs have the issue of poor solubility that restrict their oral bioavailability [33]. In addition, various anticancer therapeutics having limited permeability across the GI membrane after oral administration [34].

Gastrointestinal tract (GIT) is an extremely complicated environment concerning chemical components and physical structure. The mucus layer in the intestine is one of the important barriers to drug absorption [35]. Shorter residence times and the presence of various efflux transporters further limit the oral absorption of drugs [36]. Expulsion of drug molecules from the cell membrane by various transporters such as P-gp (P-glycoproteins), breast cancer resistant protein, MDR (multidrug resistance protein), and cytoplasmic transport proteins is responsible for drug efflux [36, 37]. MDR is prominent in enterocytes of intestinal epithelia that encodes P-gp and constitutes major drug efflux transporter responsible to expel the absorbed drug molecule outside [37]. Vinblastine, vincristine, docetaxel, paclitaxel, etoposide, and doxorubicin are common examples of anti-neoplastic molecules known as a major substrate of efflux transporter [37, 38]. In addition, pH variation, surface-active agents like bile salts, and enzymes in the Gastrointestinal tract and the liver collectively constitute the biochemical barriers for the absorption of anticancer drugs after oral administration [39]. The variation in pH condition from acidic to alkaline, along the GI tract imposes a hurdle for the drugs and nanoparticles stability. Further, surfactants in the GIT can also have a significant influence on the structural integrity of the drug-loaded nano-particulate system. Furthermore, metabolic enzymes such as Cytochrome P-450, specifically Cytochrome P3A4 in the intestinal cells and liver further limit drug absorption after oral administration [39, 40]. The oral bioavailability of a drug is a function of the amount of drug that is absorbed from the entero-hepatic circulation and the amount of drug that is available after the first pass metabolism [41]. Metabolism in the GIT or the luminal metabolism is a combined result of various digestive enzymes secreted from the pancreas which include lipases, peptidases and amylases, and the GI flora present in the lower parts of the tract. Cytochrome P450 3A family, especially the Cytochrome P 3A4, which are the common metabolizing enzymes in phase 1, are found in the intestinal absorptive cells that carry out to the metabolism of the cytotoxic drugs in the gastrointestinal wall. Glutathione-S, esterases, and transferases are major phase-II metabolizing enzymes that are said to be present in the intestine [42]. The intestinal epithelium causes low bioavailability of drugs (capecitabine) by acting as a site for metabolism [43]. The liver acts as the main site for metabolic clearance of various endogenous chemicals and xenobiotics. The first-pass metabolism is the main cause for the lower oral bioavailability of several anticancer therapeutics [44]. To further worsen the condition, if the drugs are potential substrates for cytochromes, they also act as a substrate for P-gp, which ultimately results in a substantial reduction in the total oral bioavailability of cancer chemotherapeutics (eg: docetaxel and paclitaxel).

A lipid-based drug delivery system, where the drug is dissolved by lipids or lipid-like excipients, has been identified as an attractive strategy for improving the systemic absorption of low bioavailable compounds of various therapeutic classes [45, 46]. Surfactants are used to stabilize this drug-loaded nanoparticulate system. The lipophilic nature and submicron dimension of lipid-based formulation guided for absorption through intestinal lymphatic transport for improved drug efficacy [47]. It further decreases the chances of drug toxicity as seen in the case of doxorubicin commercial product Doxil®/Caelyx® compared to Adriamycin® [48]. Indeed, among the various route of drug administration for the lipid-based formulation, the oral route remains the most popular and favored routes of administration since it is non-invasive, economical, and is less prone to side effects. The commonly used lipid-based formulation for oral administration of anti-cancer drugs include *lipid micelles, lipid-drug conjugate, solid lipid nanoparticles, liposomes, nanostructured lipid carriers,* and *self-nanoemulsifying drug delivery system (SNEDDS)*. Among the various lipid-based formulations for delivery of anti-cancer drugs, SNEDDS found to be most feasible and economical for anticancer oral therapy. In addition, advancements in the research of homolipids and heterolipids as excipients, SNEDDS formulations have gained much attention to improve the oral efficacy of poorly bioavailable cancer chemotherapeutics. They have wide compatibility with various cytotoxic drugs, surfactants, and oil system as well as easy to process and manufacture. Thereby, attracting further interest to explore SNEDDS as a drug carrier for the development of anticancer oral therapy.

SELF-NANOEMULSIFYING DRUG DELIVERY SYSTEM FOR ANTICANCER ORAL THERAPY

It is an isotropic mixture of oil, surfactants along with co-surfactants having the ability to form nanoemulsions with droplet size <200 nm upon gentle agitation following dilution with the aqueous phase [49]. The self-emulsification process is aided by the agitation provided from the motility of the intestines and stomach during digestion [49, 50]. As SNEDDS self-emulsify in the stomach and presents the drug in the form small droplets of oil, it enhances drug dissolution by providing a big interfacial region for a division of the drug between the oil and gastrointestinal (GI) fluid besides improving stability [51] as shown in Fig. (**1**). For drugs that have dissolution as the rate-limiting step for their absorption, SNEDDS enhances the bioavailability by enhancing both the amount and rate of drug absorbed and also presents the advantage of plasma concentration reproducibility. One additional advantage in using SNEDDS with oral drugs that are P-gp substrates is their ability to carry or solubilize high levels of specific (second and third generation) and nonspecific (first generation) P-gp inhibitors illustrated in Fig. (**2**). It is also reported that vegetable and animal oils used as a formulation component in the development of SNEDDS may have differential effects on particular hepatic CYP isoforms and may adjoin to the unevenness in metabolism when xenobiotics are delivered in lipid-based vehicle [52, 53]. It is a widely used drug delivery vehicle for different lipophilic anticancer therapeutics of lipophilic nature [54, 55].

The marketed product of SNEDDS of various therapeutic classes further validates its significance to solve out the biopharmaceutical challenges in oral administration of hydrophobic drugs (Table **1**). SNEDDS can enhance drug absorption in various ways. It improved the drug solubilization behavior in the intestine and modulating different drug transporter through inhibition of P-gp efflux and metabolism. It also favors additional absorption of the drug to the systemic circulation through the intestinal lymphatic transport pathway.

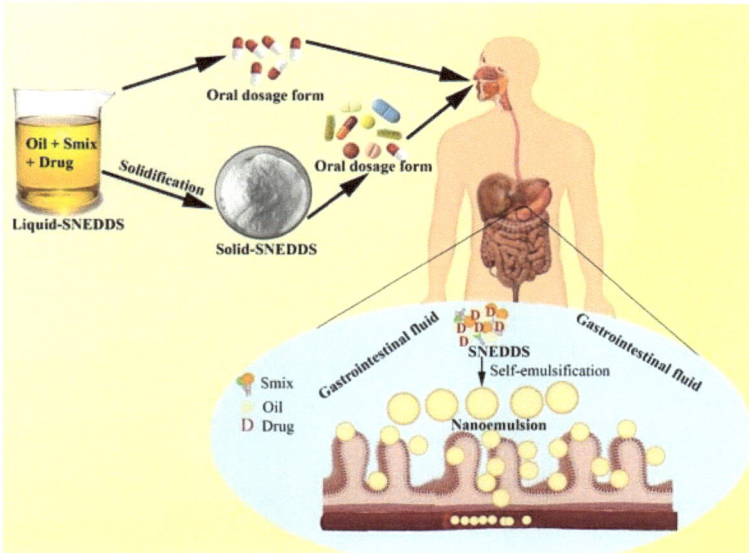

Fig. (1). Illustration showing the oral absorption of the drug through SNEDDS.

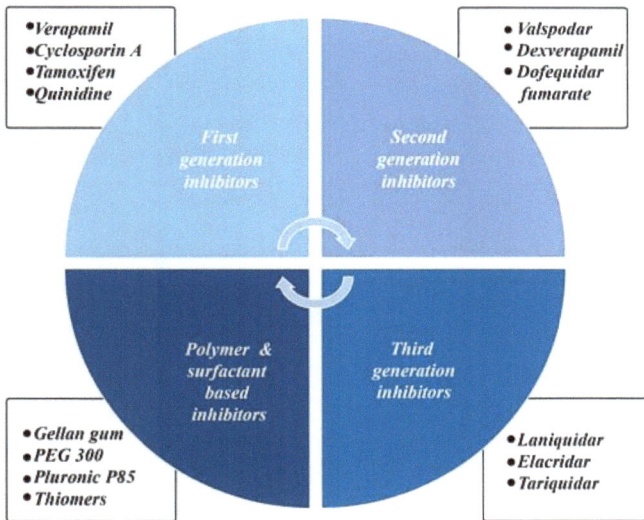

Fig. (2). Illustration showing a different class of P-gp inhibitors.

Table 1. Some of the marketed preparation of self-emulsifying drug delivery system.

Drug	TradeName/ Company	Water Solubility	Dosage Form	Excipients
Amprenavir	Agenerase® (**Glaxo Smith Kline**)	Practically insoluble	Soft gelatin capsule	TPGS, Propylene glycol, PEG 400
Cyclosporin A	Neoral® (**Novartis**)	Slightly soluble	Soft gelatin capsule	Corn oil, dl-tocopherol, Cremophor RH40, Glycerol, Ethanol, Propylene glycol
Cyclosporin A	Sandimmune® (**Novartis**)	Slightly soluble	Soft gelatin capsule	Labrafil M-2125 CS, Corn oil, Ethanol, Glycerol
Cyclosporin A	Gengraf® (**Abbott**)	Slightly soluble	Hard gelatin capsule	Cremophor EL, Ethanol, Propylene glycol, Polysorbate 80
Isotretinoin	Accutane® (**Roche**)	Practically insoluble	Soft gelatin capsule	Hydrogenated soybean oil flakes, Beeswax, Soybean oil, hydrogenated vegetable oils, BHA
Ritonavir	Norvir® (**Abbott**)	Practically insoluble	Soft gelatin capsule	Oleic acid, Cremophor EL, Ethanol, BHT
Saquinavir	Fortovase® (**Roche**)	Slightly soluble	Soft gelatin capsule	Medium-chain mono- and diglycerides, dl-α-tocopherol, Povidone
Fenofibrate	Fenogal® (**Genus**)	Practically insoluble	Hard gelatin capsule	Gelucire 44/14, hydrogenated vegetable oil, PEG-20,000, HPC
Lopinavir and ritonavir	Kaletra® (**Abbott**)	Practically insoluble	Soft gelatin capsule	Oleic acid, Propylene glycol, Cremophor EL
Tipranavir	Aptivus® (**BoehringerIngelheim**)	Slightly soluble	Soft gelatin capsule	Medium-chain mono-diglycerides, Cremophor EL, propylene glycol, Ethanol

Contemporary Research and Application

SNEDDS is the highly developed strategy of emulsion dependent drug delivery systems and it is based on the physiological fluids for *in-situ* nanoemulsion formation [56]. The advancement in the field of biocompatible lipid and their derivatives in addition to recent findings on pharmaceutical excipients such as oil, surfactants, co-surfactants having P-gp modulating potential further extend the interest in SNEDDS for oral delivery of cytotoxic drugs. The contemporary research in the area of SNEDDS associated with its *in vitro* as well as *in vivo* results after oral administration of cancer therapeutics is briefly discussed below and summarized in Table **2**.

Table 2. Self-emulsifying drug delivery system exploited to enhance the oral efficacy of cancer chemotherapeutics.

S.No.	Cancer Chemotherapeutics	Outcome of the Investigation	Ref.
1.	Docetaxel	SNEDDS increased oral bioavailability of docetaxel through the co-delivery of cyclosporine A	[57]
2.	Etoposide (VP-16)	SNEDDS resulted 6.4 fold increase in $AUC_{0 \to t}$ of VP-16	[58]
3.	Cisplatin	SNEDDS improved therapeutic activity and minimized cisplatin related nephrotoxicity	[60]
4.	Paclitaxel	SNEDDS improved the oral bioavailability and cytotoxic activity of paclitaxel by co-delivery of curcumin	[61]
5.	Paclitaxel	Paclitaxel loaded SNEDDS using excipients with P-gp modulating characteristics was developed and characterize with droplet size <100 nm	[53]
6.	Etoposide	Etoposide loaded SNEDDS was developed using P-gp inhibitory surfactants and improved the drug cellular uptake.	[64]
7.	Irinotecan	Irinotecan loaded SNEDDS exhibited deeper penetration of drug in the intestine, observed by confocal laser scanning microscopy	[66]
8.	Methotrexate	Methotrexate with β-cyclodextrin as inclusion complex was developed into SNEDDS and demonstrated 1.57-fold enhancement in oral bioavailability.	[69]
9.	Docetaxel	The presence of curcumin did not reduce the systemic clearance and improved oral bioavailability due to the suppression of Cyp-3A and P-gp.	[70]
10.	Etoposide	Etoposide-phospholipid complex (EPC) was produced and converted to SNEDDS which ultimately cause a significant improvement in oral bioavailability	[73]
11.	9-nitrocamptothecin	9-nitrocamptothecin loaded SNEDDS provided proof-of-concept as a potential drug delivery system to enhance the oral bioavailability and antitumor properties of lipophilic anticancer drugs.	[76]
12.	BCNU	BCNU loaded SNEDDS delayed the rate of drug degradation and increased cell cytotoxicity.	[79]

Recently, Cui *et al.* have developed SNEDDS formulation for co-delivery of docetaxel and cyclosporine A after oral administration. The developed formulation successfully achieved the improvement in the oral bioavailability of docetaxel due to effective inhibition of P-gp efflux and P450 enzyme metabolism by the cyclosporine A [57]. Also, Khalid *et al.* have explored the ability of SNEDDS to increase bioavailability after oral administration etoposide (VP-16) as a model drug [58]. It was found that $AUC_{0 \to t}$ of VP-16 containing SNEDDS is 6.4-fold greater than VP-16 drug suspension. Similarly, Shakeel *et al.* designed vanillin loaded SNEDDS to improve its antioxidant and cytotoxic potential [59].

The *in vitro* activity was evaluated using colorectal human cancer cells (HT-29) and found to be a 2-fold increase in efficacy compared to free vanillin. In another investigation, Osman *et al.* have investigated the potential of cisplatin loaded SNEDDS to improve its therapeutic activity and reduction in cisplatin related nephrotoxicity [60]. Cisplatin loaded SNEDDS resulted in an increase in mean survival time of EAC tumor-bearing mice in comparison to free cisplatin and retained the serum urea, creatinine, and TAC level of animal to normal level. Moreover, Sandhu *et al.* have explored the potential of SNEDDS exploiting polyunsaturated fatty acids as oil phase to increase the oral bioavailability and cytotoxic activity of paclitaxel by co-delivery of curcumin as well [61]. It was found that the co-delivery strategy of paclitaxel with curcumin exploiting SNEDDS as a delivery vehicle remarkably increase the extent of oral absorption of paclitaxel. Certain formulation excipients of SNEDDS has the potential to influence the P-gp efflux transporter for better absorption of substrate drug. Ahmad *et al.* utilizing this concept and developed paclitaxel loaded SNEDDS using excipients with P-glycoprotein (P-gp) modulating characteristics [53]. In another investigation, Ahmad *et al.* demonstrated and optimize SNEDDS exploiting Box–Behnken experimental design for oral administration of poorly soluble drugs like paclitaxel as a model drug [55]. Moreover, Heshmati *et al.* demonstrated the digestion of four indirubin-3'-oxime 2,3-dihydroxypropyl ether (E804) loaded SNEDDS by the assessment of dynamic lipolysis and reported their improved bioavailability [62]. Patel *et al.* produced medium-chain triglyceride containing SNEDDS loaded with cytotoxic drugs [63]. SNEDDS showed improved precipitation kinetic profile, superior drug loading with minor hemolysis, and histamine liberation than marketed formulation.

Etoposide is a substrate for P-gp transporter and cytochrome P450 3A (CYP3A), having poor water-solubility. Zhong *et al.* have enhanced the bioavailability of etoposide by formulating SNEDDS consist of CYP-3A and P-gp inhibitory surfactants like Cremophor EL and Cremophor RH40, Polysorbate-80 [64]. Similarly, Akhter *et al.* studied the possibility of etoposide containing SNEDDS for increased bioavailability exploiting modulation of P-gp transporter upon oral administration [65]. In another investigation, Negi *et al.* prepared SNEDDS of Irinotecan by using P-gp modulatory excipients [66]. The deeper penetration of drug in the intestine was investigated by confocal laser scanning microscopy and demonstrated an improved drug penetration. SNEDDS is an important approach to increase the solubility and oral bioavailability. Heshmati *et al.* produced and assessed a SNEDDS consisting of E804 for increasing its solubility and bioavailability [67]. Quan *et al.* designed SNEDDS for the oral delivery of docetaxel as an option to marketed docetaxel-loaded injectable products [68]. In another study, an inclusion complex of methotrexate with β-cyclodextrin was produced by Bourkaib *et al.* as to reduce its photosensitivity and increase its aqueous solubility [69]. Yan *et al.* studied the outcomes of curcumin SNEDDS on the oral pharmacokinetics of docetaxel in rats [70]. Single-dose studies of oral delivery showed Cmax and AUC to be significantly improved. He *et al.*, to handle the problems of low water solubility of teniposide, the contribution of toxic surfactant in its injection, and the poor stability during infusion, produced a cremophor-free teniposide loaded SNEDDS [71]. Zhang *et al.* produced and assessed a folate-modified SNEDDS to increase the solubility of curcumin and its delivery to the colon [72]. Moreover, Wu *et al.* produced a new phospholipid complex SNEDDS to increase the bioavailability of oral etoposide [73]. Etoposide-phospholipid complex (EPC) was produced by reacting etoposide and phospholipid in tetrahydrofuran. The synergistic effect of phospholipid complex and SNEDDS assisted in the increased bioavailability of etoposide. In another study, Wu *et al.* produced SNEDDS of curcumin to surmount the limitations like poor solubility, low stability in aqueous solution, and *in vivo* low bioavailability [74].

Cremophore free nonionic self-emulsifying oil-in-water (O/W) system was composed by Lo *et al.* as drug delivery carriers for anticancer drugs [75]. In another investigation, Lu *et al.* prepared 9-nitrocamptothecin loaded SNEDDS [76]. It was observed that the $AUC_{0 \rightarrow 8h}$ values of different preparations of 9-nitrocamptothecin following oral delivery showed significant improvement for SNEDDS in comparison to 9-nitrocamptothecin solution and 9-nitrocamptothecin suspension. However, Quan *et al.* prepared puerarin containing SNEDDS and assessed its absolute bioavailability [77]. Similarly, Cui *et al.* produced and characterized SNEDDS of Pueraria lobata isoflavone to increase its bioavailability [78]. In another investigation, Chae *et al.* produced SNEDDS for improved stability of BCNU (1,3-bis(2-chloroethyl)-1-nitrosourea) [79]. All of the data suggested that SNEDDS significantly enhanced stability. Taha *et al.* worked on SNEDDS of all-trans-retinol acetate and optimized the formulation through a 3-factorial 3-level Box-Behnken design [80]. The experimental data and the response from created equations were in close agreement indicating that Box-Behnken design is a good approach to optimize the SNEDDS.

Recent Progress and Advancement

The conventional preparation of SNEDDS requires the dissolution of drugs in oil and fusing with an optimal solubilizing agent. SNEDDS prepared by these methods, however, have shown disadvantages such as low stability, low drug loading, portability, and increasing costs of production. The usage of irreversible drugs and excipients is also challenging [81]. Huge concentrations of surfactants which are between 30-60% causes GI irritation. Even with their advantages, one has to overcome these challenges to make SNEDDS an acceptable dosage form. The compatibility of SNEDDS with capsule shells is also of prime importance since alcohol and other co-solvents of volatile nature evaporate into the capsule shells thereby causing drug precipitation [82]. Solidification remains as a feasible approach for stabilizing the SNEDDS and offers several advantages such as a) reduction in the administration volume, b) precision dosing, c) easy storage and transfer, and d) improved patient compliance [83, 84].

To deal with the challenges associated with conventional self-emulsifying (SE) formulation, solid SE systems have been investigated. This formulation strategy involves the solidification of liquid SE systems into different solid dosage forms [85]. The liquid-SNEDDS can be transformed into a solid dosage form without disturbing self-emulsification performance and release profile of therapeutics. Self-emulsification occurs in GIT by the liberated content. Thus, solid-SNEDDS unite the benefits of SNEDDS (like improved solubility and bioavailability) and solid dosage forms (like great stability and reproducibility, compact form, convenience in handling, and portability, as well as improved patient compliance) [86]. Knowing the benefits of solid dosage forms, solid-SNDDS have been widely studied in recent years, as they often correspond to more effective options to conventional liquid-SEDDS. From the dosage forms view, solid-SNEDDS mean solid dosage forms with self-emulsification properties. Solid-SNEDDS focus on the integration of liquid/semisolid SE components into powders/nanoparticles by various solidification techniques.

Solidification Technique Transforming SNEDDS into Solid Dosage Forms

Solid-SNEDDSs are produced from liquid/semisolid SNEDDS majorly by using the solidification techniques like adsorption on solid carriers [87], spray drying [88], lyophilization [89] and melt extrusion/spheronization technology [90]. Such powders/nanoparticles, that are known as SE nanoparticles/dry emulsions/solid dispersions, are normally further processed into other solid SE dosage forms or, optionally, packed into capsules. Depending on the kinds and levels of concentration of each of the excipient, SNEDDS (prepared typically without co-solvents) can re-disperse easily to form white and turbid emulsions with the droplet size range of greater than 100 nm. SNEDDS, on the other hand, can form thermodynamically stable emulsions which are clear to translucent with their droplet size ranging below 100 nm [91]. For SNEDDS containing volatile substances like ethanol or transcutol as co-solvents, suitable care must be taken when selecting solid carriers and the solidification technique to be employed, because formulating under raised temperatures (such as spray drying) and reduced pressures (such as freeze-drying) may create a challenge in preserving the volatile components [92].

Challenges with Solidification Techniques

There are various problems related to solidification technologies [86]. It may include the quantity and nature of solidifying excipients that may influence drug release as well as absorption. It may cause phase separation on reconstitution or drug degradation during the solidification process. Also, solidification through spray drying might result in blockage of the spraying nozzle. Variation in drug content uniformity and chances of residual solvent while granulation is another challenge associated with solidification technologies.

Strategies to Overcome the Challenges Associated with Solidification Techniques

Various approaches to surmount the problems related to solidification technologies are discussed below:

• Gelled SNEDDS is an approach to decrease the quantity of solidifying excipients needed for conversion of SNEDDS to solid dosage forms. Colloidal silicon dioxide (Aerosil 200) is a widely used gelling agent that decreasing the quantity of solidifying excipients required for solidification as well as sustained/prolonged the drug release [93].
• Polyoxyethylene (POE) may employ as an inert solid carrier to develop solid-SNEDDS by a simple fusion method. Ahmad *et al.* have investigated the potential of solid-SNEDDS to improve the oral absorption of paclitaxel employing POE as a solidifying agent for SNEDDS [94].
• To prevent the phase separation of capsule dosage forms containing liquid-SNEDDS in the GI environment should consist of sodium dodecyl sulfate to observe the enhancement in oral absorption of pay-load [95]. In addition, HPMC or other polymers may use along with liquid-SNEDDS to avoid the drug precipitation and sustaining a supersaturated state in the *in vivo* system [96]. Further, such a delivery approach decreases the possibility of GI-related untoward effect because of using a decreased quantity of surfactant.
• Self-emulsifying (SE) solid dispersions composed of SE excipients such as Gelucire 44/14, Gelucire150/02, Labrasol, Transcutol, and TPGS significantly enhance the absorption of drugs with low solubility compared to PEG solid dispersions [97, 98]. It easily packed into hard gelatin capsules in the molten state, thereby avoiding the requirement of milling and blending before filling.

CONCLUDING REMARKS

SNEDDS is exploited as an important tool to enhance the oral efficacy of anticancer therapeutics. The reduction of size to submicron range provides a greater surface area for enhanced dissolution and permeation across biological barriers. In addition, depending on widespread preclinical and clinical research, the viability of the oral route of administration of cancer chemotherapeutics in cancer patients by concomitant administration of P-glycoprotein inhibitor is seen. These P-gp inhibitors, generally, are either first-generation, second, or third generation. All these are known to exhibit toxicity or pharmacological interactions. However, nowadays, pharmacological inactive pharmaceutical excipients used in SNEDDS as formulation components have been identified to inhibit P-gp efflux pumps. Therefore, concurrent employment of SNEDDS with P-gp modulating formulation components appears to be a better strategy for oral administration of cancer chemotherapeutics. The detailed clinical investigation required further in designing a formulation of self-emulsifying nature that readily encapsulates the therapeutics in nanocarrier immediately when comes in contact with GI fluid. Furthermore, the systematic study for the effect of formulation factors is observed by utilizing the Quality-by-Design (QbD) approach to understand the factors and their interaction by a desired set of experiments.

CONSENT FOR PUBLICATION

Not applicable.

CONFLICT OF INTEREST

The author confirms that this chapter contents have no conflict of interest.

ACKNOWLEDGEMENTS

Declared none.

LIST OF ABBREVIATIONS

AUC	Area under the curve
BCNU	1,3-bis(2-chloroethyl)-1-nitrosourea
BHA	Butylated hydroxyanisole
BHT	Butylated hydroxytoluene
CYP3A	Cytochrome P450 3A
EPC	Etoposide-phospholipid complex
GI	Gastrointestinal
GIT	Gastrointestinal tract

HPMC	Hydroxypropyl methylcellulose
MDR	Multidrug resistance protein
O/W	Oil-in-water
PEG	Polyethylene glycol
P-gp	P-glycoproteins
POE	Polyoxyethylene
QbD	Quality-by-Design
SE	Self-emulsifying
SNEDDS	Self-nanoemulsifying drug delivery system
TPGS	D -α-Tocopherol polyethylene glycol 1000 succinate

REFERENCES

[1]   Luo J, Solimini NL, Elledge SJ. Principles of cancer therapy: oncogene and non-oncogene addiction. Cell 2009; 136(5): 823-37.
[http://dx.doi.org/10.1016/j.cell.2009.02.024] [PMID: 19269363]

[2]   WHO 2018: IARC (International Agency for Research on Cancer). Available from: https://www.who.int/cancer/PRGlobocanFinal.pdf

[3]   Khan MA, Jain VK, Rizwanullah M, Ahmad J, Jain K. PI3K/AKT/mTOR pathway inhibitors in triple-negative breast cancer: a review on drug discovery and future challenges. Drug Discov Today 2019; 24(11): 2181-91.
[http://dx.doi.org/10.1016/j.drudis.2019.09.001] [PMID: 31520748]

[4]   Aggarwal S. Targeted cancer therapies. Nat Rev Drug Discov 2010; 9(6): 427-8.
[http://dx.doi.org/10.1038/nrd3186] [PMID: 20514063]

[5]   Prakash S, Malhotra M, Shao W, Tomaro-Duchesneau C, Abbasi S. Polymeric nanohybrids and functionalized carbon nanotubes as drug delivery carriers for cancer therapy. Adv Drug Deliv Rev 2011; 63(14-15): 1340-51.
[http://dx.doi.org/10.1016/j.addr.2011.06.013] [PMID: 21756952]

[6]   Ahmad J, Akhter S, Rizwanullah M, *et al.* Nanotechnology-based inhalation treatments for lung cancer: state of the art. Nanotechnol Sci Appl 2015; 8: 55-66.
[PMID: 26640374]

[7]   Ewesuedo RB, Ratain MJ. Principles of Cancer Chemotherapy. In: Vokes EE, Golomb HM, Eds. Oncologic Therapies. Berlin: Springer 2003; 19-66.
[http://dx.doi.org/10.1007/978-3-642-55780-4_3]

[8]   Lønning PE. Study of suboptimum treatment response: lessons from breast cancer. Lancet Oncol 2003; 4(3): 177-85.
[http://dx.doi.org/10.1016/S1470-2045(03)01022-2] [PMID: 12623363]

[9]   Ratain MJ, Mick R. Principles of pharmacokinetic and pharmacodynamics. In: Schilsky, RL, Milano, GA, Ratain, MJ, Eds. Principles of antineoplastic drug development and pharmacology, New York: Marcel Dekker 1996; 123-42.

[10]   Feng SS, Chien S. Chemotherapeutic engineering: application and further development of chemical engineering principles for chemotherapy of cancer and other diseases. Chem Eng Sci 2003; 58: 4087-114.
[http://dx.doi.org/10.1016/S0009-2509(03)00234-3]

[11] O'Neill VJ, Twelves CJ. Oral cancer treatment: developments in chemotherapy and beyond. Br J Cancer 2002; 87(9): 933-7.
[http://dx.doi.org/10.1038/sj.bjc.6600591] [PMID: 12434279]

[12] Khandelwal N, Duncan I, Ahmed T, Rubinstein E, Pegus C. Oral chemotherapy program improves adherence and reduces medication wastage and hospital admissions. J Natl Compr Canc Netw 2012; 10(5): 618-25.
[http://dx.doi.org/10.6004/jnccn.2012.0063] [PMID: 22570292]

[13] Roop JC, Wu HS. Current practice patterns for oral chemotherapy: results of a national survey. Oncol Nurs Forum 2014; 41(2): 185-94.
[http://dx.doi.org/10.1188/14.ONF.41-02AP] [PMID: 24370897]

[14] Rizwanullah M, Ahmad J, Amin S, Mishra A, Ain MR, Rahman M. Polymer-lipid hybrid systems: scope of intravenous-to-oral switch in cancer chemotherapy. Curr Nanomed 2020; 10: 1-13.
[http://dx.doi.org/10.2174/2468187309666190514083508].

[15] Ruddy K, Mayer E, Partridge A. Patient adherence and persistence with oral anticancer treatment. CA Cancer J Clin 2009; 59(1): 56-66.
[http://dx.doi.org/10.3322/caac.20004] [PMID: 19147869]

[16] Weingart SN, Brown E, Bach PB, et al. NCCN task force report: oral chemotherapy. J Natl Compr Canc Netw 2008; 6 (Suppl. 3): S1-S14.
[http://dx.doi.org/10.6004/jnccn.2008.2003] [PMID: 18377852]

[17] Given BA, Spoelstra SL, Grant M. The challenges of oral agents as antineoplastic treatments. Semin Oncol Nurs 2011; 27(2): 93-103.
[http://dx.doi.org/10.1016/j.soncn.2011.02.003] [PMID: 21514479]

[18] Liu G, Franssen E, Fitch MI, Warner E. Patient preferences for oral *versus* intravenous palliative chemotherapy. J Clin Oncol 1997; 15(1): 110-5.
[http://dx.doi.org/10.1200/JCO.1997.15.1.110] [PMID: 8996131]

[19] Wojtacki J, Wiraszka R, Rolka-Stempniewicz G, et al. Breast cancer patient's preferences for oral *versus* intravenous second-line anticancer therapy. Eur J Cancer 2006; 4(suppl 2): 159-60.

[20] Paley M, Love N, Carlson R, et al. Preferences for oral, parenteral antitumor therapy: a survey of 260 patients with metastatic breast cancer. Proc Am Soc Clin Oncol 2005; 23: 619.
[http://dx.doi.org/10.1200/jco.2005.23.16_suppl.619]

[21] Aisner J. Overview of the changing paradigm in cancer treatment: oral chemotherapy. Am J Health Syst Pharm 2007; 64(9) (Suppl. 5): S4-7.
[http://dx.doi.org/10.2146/ajhp070035] [PMID: 17468157]

[22] Ahmad J, Kohli K, Mir SR, Amin S. Lipid based nanocarriers for oral delivery of cancer chemotherapeutics: an insight in the intestinal lymphatic transport. Drug Deliv Lett 2013; 3(1): 38-46.
[http://dx.doi.org/10.2174/2210304x11303010006]

[23] Ahmad J, Amin S, Rahman M, et al. Solid matrix based lipidic nanoparticles in oral cancer chemotherapy: Applications and pharmacokinetics. Curr Drug Metab 2015; 16(8): 633-44.
[http://dx.doi.org/10.2174/1389200216666150812122128] [PMID: 26264206]

[24] Banna GL, Collovà E, Gebbia V, et al. Anticancer oral therapy: emerging related issues. Cancer Treat Rev 2010; 36(8): 595-605.
[http://dx.doi.org/10.1016/j.ctrv.2010.04.005] [PMID: 20570443]

[25] Mazzaferro S, Bouchemal K, Ponchel G. Oral delivery of anticancer drugs I: general considerations. Drug Discov Today 2013; 18(1-2): 25-34.
[http://dx.doi.org/10.1016/j.drudis.2012.08.004] [PMID: 22951365]

[26] Harshita , Barkat MA, Rizwanullah M, et al. Paclitaxel-loaded nanolipidic carriers with improved oral bioavailability and anticancer activity against human liver carcinoma. AAPS PharmSciTech 2019;

20(2): 87.
[http://dx.doi.org/10.1208/s12249-019-1304-4] [PMID: 30675689]

[27]   Koolen SL, Beijnen JH, Schellens JH. Intravenous-to-oral switch in anticancer chemotherapy: a focus on docetaxel and paclitaxel. Clin Pharmacol Ther 2010; 87(1): 126-9.
[http://dx.doi.org/10.1038/clpt.2009.233] [PMID: 19924122]

[28]   Soni K, Rizwanullah M, Kohli K. Development and optimization of sulforaphane-loaded nanostructured lipid carriers by the Box-Behnken design for improved oral efficacy against cancer: *in vitro*, *ex vivo* and *in vivo* assessments. Artif Cells Nanomed Biotechnol 2018; 46(sup1): 15-31.
[http://dx.doi.org/10.1080/21691401.2017.1408124]

[29]   Lipinski CA. Drug-like properties and the causes of poor solubility and poor permeability. J Pharmacol Toxicol Methods 2000; 44(1): 235-49.
[http://dx.doi.org/10.1016/S1056-8719(00)00107-6] [PMID: 11274893]

[30]   Ahmad J, Singhal M, Amin S, *et al.* Bile salt stabilized vesicles (Bilosomes): A novel nano-pharmaceutical design for oral delivery of proteins and peptides. Curr Pharm Des 2017; 23(11): 1575-88.
[http://dx.doi.org/10.2174/1381612823666170124111142] [PMID: 28120725]

[31]   Rabanel JM, Aoun V, Elkin I, Mokhtar M, Hildgen P. Drug-loaded nanocarriers: passive targeting and crossing of biological barriers. Curr Med Chem 2012; 19(19): 3070-102.
[http://dx.doi.org/10.2174/092986712800784702] [PMID: 22612696]

[32]   Luo C, Sun J, Du Y, He Z. Emerging integrated nanohybrid drug delivery systems to facilitate the intravenous-to-oral switch in cancer chemotherapy. J Control Release 2014; 176: 94-103.
[http://dx.doi.org/10.1016/j.jconrel.2013.12.030] [PMID: 24389337]

[33]   Sugano K. Fraction of a dose absorbed estimation for structurally diverse low solubility compounds. Int J Pharm 2011; 405(1-2): 79-89.
[http://dx.doi.org/10.1016/j.ijpharm.2010.11.049] [PMID: 21134428]

[34]   Yee S. *in vitro* permeability across Caco-2 cells (colonic) can predict *in vivo* (small intestinal) absorption in man--fact or myth. Pharm Res 1997; 14(6): 763-6.
[http://dx.doi.org/10.1023/A:1012102522787] [PMID: 9210194]

[35]   Doherty MM, Charman WN. The mucosa of the small intestine: how clinically relevant as an organ of drug metabolism? Clin Pharmacokinet 2002; 41(4): 235-53.
[http://dx.doi.org/10.2165/00003088-200241040-00001] [PMID: 11978143]

[36]   Szakács G, Váradi A, Ozvegy-Laczka C, Sarkadi B. The role of ABC transporters in drug absorption, distribution, metabolism, excretion and toxicity (ADME-Tox). Drug Discov Today 2008; 13(9-10): 379-93.
[http://dx.doi.org/10.1016/j.drudis.2007.12.010] [PMID: 18468555]

[37]   Breedveld P, Beijnen JH, Schellens JH. Use of P-glycoprotein and BCRP inhibitors to improve oral bioavailability and CNS penetration of anticancer drugs. Trends Pharmacol Sci 2006; 27(1): 17-24.
[http://dx.doi.org/10.1016/j.tips.2005.11.009] [PMID: 16337012]

[38]   Ambudkar SV, Ramachandra M, Cardarelli CO, Pastan I, Gottesman MM. Modulation of human P-glycoprotein ATPase activity by interaction between overlapping substrate-binding sites. Proc Annu Meet Am Assoc Cancer Res 1996; 325.

[39]   Agoram B, Woltosz WS, Bolger MB. Predicting the impact of physiological and biochemical processes on oral drug bioavailability. Adv Drug Deliv Rev 2001; 50 (Suppl. 1): S41-67.
[http://dx.doi.org/10.1016/S0169-409X(01)00179-X] [PMID: 11576695]

[40]   van Herwaarden AE, van Waterschoot RA, Schinkel AH. How important is intestinal cytochrome P450 3A metabolism? Trends Pharmacol Sci 2009; 30(5): 223-7.
[http://dx.doi.org/10.1016/j.tips.2009.02.003] [PMID: 19328560]

[41]   Wu CY, Benet LZ, Hebert MF, *et al.* Differentiation of absorption and first-pass gut and hepatic

metabolism in humans: studies with cyclosporine. Clin Pharmacol Ther 1995; 58(5): 492-7.
[http://dx.doi.org/10.1016/0009-9236(95)90168-X] [PMID: 7586942]

[42]   Shen DD, Kunze KL, Thummel KE. Enzyme-catalyzed processes of first-pass hepatic and intestinal drug extraction. Adv Drug Deliv Rev 1997; 27(2-3): 99-127.
[http://dx.doi.org/10.1016/S0169-409X(97)00039-2] [PMID: 10837554]

[43]   Tabata T, Katoh M, Tokudome S, Nakajima M, Yokoi T. Identification of the cytosolic carboxylesterase catalyzing the 5'-deoxy-5-fluorocytidine formation from capecitabine in human liver. Drug Metab Dispos 2004; 32(10): 1103-10.
[http://dx.doi.org/10.1124/dmd.104.000554] [PMID: 15269188]

[44]   Shin SC, Choi JS, Li X. Enhanced bioavailability of tamoxifen after oral administration of tamoxifen with quercetin in rats. Int J Pharm 2006; 313(1-2): 144-9.
[http://dx.doi.org/10.1016/j.ijpharm.2006.01.028] [PMID: 16516418]

[45]   Hauss DJ. Oral lipid-based formulations. Adv Drug Deliv Rev 2007; 59(7): 667-76.
[http://dx.doi.org/10.1016/j.addr.2007.05.006] [PMID: 17618704]

[46]   Fatouros DG, Karpf DM, Nielsen FS, Mullertz A. Clinical studies with oral lipid based formulations of poorly soluble compounds. Ther Clin Risk Manag 2007; 3(4): 591-604.
[PMID: 18472981]

[47]   Akhter MH, Rizwanullah M, Ahmad J, Ahsan MJ, Mujtaba MA, Amin S. Nanocarriers in advanced drug targeting: setting novel paradigm in cancer therapeutics. Artif Cells Nanomed Biotechnol 2018; 46(5): 873-84.
[http://dx.doi.org/10.1080/21691401.2017.1366333] [PMID: 28830262]

[48]   O'Brien ME, Wigler N, Inbar M, *et al.* CAELYX Breast Cancer Study Group. Reduced cardiotoxicity and comparable efficacy in a phase III trial of pegylated liposomal doxorubicin HCl (CAELYX/Doxil) *versus* conventional doxorubicin for first-line treatment of metastatic breast cancer. Ann Oncol 2004; 15(3): 440-9.
[http://dx.doi.org/10.1093/annonc/mdh097] [PMID: 14998846]

[49]   Ahmad J, Kohli K, Mir SR, Amin S. Formulation of self-nanoemulsifying drug delivery system for telmisartan with improved dissolution and oral bioavailability. J Dispers Sci Technol 2011; 32(7): 958-68.
[http://dx.doi.org/10.1080/01932691.2010.488511]

[50]   Jing-ling T, Jin S, Zhong-Gui H. Self-Emulsifying Drug Delivery Systems: Strategy for Improving Oral Delivery of Poorly Soluble Drugs. Curr Drug Ther 2007; 2: 85-93.
[http://dx.doi.org/10.2174/157488507779422400]

[51]   Pouton CW. Lipid formulations for oral administration of drugs: non-emulsifying, self-emulsifying and 'self-microemulsifying' drug delivery systems. Eur J Pharm Sci 2000; 11 (Suppl. 2): S93-8.
[http://dx.doi.org/10.1016/S0928-0987(00)00167-6] [PMID: 11033431]

[52]   Brunner LJ, Bai S. Effect of dietary oil intake on hepatic cytochrome P450 activity in the rat. J Pharm Sci 2000; 89(8): 1022-7.
[http://dx.doi.org/10.1002/1520-6017(200008)89:8<1022::AID-JPS6>3.0.CO;2-O] [PMID: 10906725]

[53]   Ahmad J, Mir SR, Kohli K, Amin S. Quality by design approach for self nanoemulsifying system of paclitaxel. Sci Adv Mater 2014; 6(8): 1778-91.
[http://dx.doi.org/10.1166/sam.2014.1884]

[54]   Akhtartavan S, Karimi M, Karimian K, Azarpira N, Khatami M, Heli H. Evaluation of a self-nanoemulsifying docetaxel delivery system. Biomed Pharmacother 2019; 109: 2427-33.
[http://dx.doi.org/10.1016/j.biopha.2018.11.110] [PMID: 30551502]

[55]   Ahmad J, Mir SR, Kohli K, Amin S. Effect of oil and co-surfactant on the formation of Solutol HS 15 based colloidal drug carrier by Box–Behnken statistical design. Colloids Surf A Physicochem Eng Asp 2014; 453: 68-77.

[http://dx.doi.org/10.1016/j.colsurfa.2014.04.008]

[56] Kohli K, Chopra S, Dhar D, Arora S, Khar RK. Self-emulsifying drug delivery systems: an approach to enhance oral bioavailability. Drug Discov Today 2010; 15(21-22): 958-65.
[http://dx.doi.org/10.1016/j.drudis.2010.08.007] [PMID: 20727418]

[57] Cui W, Zhao H, Wang C, *et al.* Co-encapsulation of docetaxel and cyclosporin A into SNEDDS to promote oral cancer chemotherapy. Drug Deliv 2019; 26(1): 542-50.
[http://dx.doi.org/10.1080/10717544.2019.1616237] [PMID: 31090467]

[58] Khalid N, Sarfraz M, Arafat M, Akhtar M, Löbenberg R, Ur Rehman N. Nano-sized droplets of self-emulsifying system for enhancing oral bioavailability of chemotherapeutic agent VP-16 in rats: A nano lipid carrier for BCS class IV drugs. J Pharm Pharm Sci 2018; 21(1): 398-408.
[http://dx.doi.org/10.18433/jpps30097] [PMID: 30365396]

[59] Shakeel F, Haq N, Raish M, Siddiqui NA, Alanazi FK, Alsarra IA. Antioxidant and cytotoxic effects of vanillin *via* eucalyptus oil containing self-nanoemulsifying drug delivery system. J Mol Liq 2016; 218: 233-9.
[http://dx.doi.org/10.1016/j.molliq.2016.02.077]

[60] Osman AM, Al-Kreathy HM, Al-Zahrani A, *et al.* Enhancement of Efficacy and Reduced Toxicity of Cisplatin Through Self Nanoemulsifying Drug Delivery System (SNEDDS). Int J Pharmacol 2017; 13(3): 292-302.
[http://dx.doi.org/10.3923/ijp.2017.292.302]

[61] Sandhu PS, Beg S, Mehta F, Singh B, Trivedi P. Novel dietary lipid-based self-nanoemulsifying drug delivery systems of paclitaxel with p-gp inhibitor: implications on cytotoxicity and biopharmaceutical performance. Expert Opin Drug Deliv 2015; 12(11): 1809-22.
[http://dx.doi.org/10.1517/17425247.2015.1060219] [PMID: 26144859]

[62] Heshmati N, Cheng X, Dapat E, *et al. in vitro* and *in vivo* evaluations of the performance of an indirubin derivative, formulated in four different self-emulsifying drug delivery systems. J Pharm Pharmacol 2014; 66(11): 1567-75.
[http://dx.doi.org/10.1111/jphp.12286] [PMID: 24961657]

[63] Patel K, Patil A, Mehta M, Gota V, Vavia P. Medium chain triglyceride (MCT) rich, paclitaxel loaded self nanoemulsifying preconcentrate (PSNP): a safe and efficacious alternative to Taxol. J Biomed Nanotechnol 2013; 9(12): 1996-2006.
[http://dx.doi.org/10.1166/jbn.2013.1710] [PMID: 24266255]

[64] Zhao G, Huang J, Xue K, Si L, Li G. Enhanced intestinal absorption of etoposide by self-microemulsifying drug delivery systems: roles of P-glycoprotein and cytochrome P450 3A inhibition. Eur J Pharm Sci 2013; 50(3-4): 429-39.
[http://dx.doi.org/10.1016/j.ejps.2013.08.016] [PMID: 23981337]

[65] Akhtar N, Talegaonkar S, Khar RK, Jaggi M. Self-nanoemulsifying lipid carrier system for enhancement of oral bioavailability of etoposide by P-glycoprotein modulation: *in vitro* cell line and *in vivo* pharmacokinetic investigation. J Biomed Nanotechnol 2013; 9(7): 1216-29.
[http://dx.doi.org/10.1166/jbn.2013.1613] [PMID: 23909136]

[66] Negi LM, Tariq M, Talegaonkar S. Nano scale self-emulsifying oil based carrier system for improved oral bioavailability of camptothecin derivative by P-Glycoprotein modulation. Colloids Surf B Biointerfaces 2013; 111: 346-53.
[http://dx.doi.org/10.1016/j.colsurfb.2013.06.001] [PMID: 23850745]

[67] Heshmati N, Cheng X, Eisenbrand G, Fricker G. Enhancement of oral bioavailability of E804 by self-nanoemulsifying drug delivery system (SNEDDS) in rats. J Pharm Sci 2013; 102(10): 3792-9.
[http://dx.doi.org/10.1002/jps.23696] [PMID: 23934779]

[68] Quan Q, Kim DW, Marasini N, *et al.* Physicochemical characterization and in vivo evaluation of solid self-nanoemulsifying drug delivery system for oral administration of docetaxel. J Microencapsul 2013; 30(4): 307-14.

[http://dx.doi.org/10.3109/02652048.2012.726280] [PMID: 23101936]

[69]   Bourkaib N, Zhou J, Yao J, Fang Z, Mezghrani O. Combination of β-cyclodextrin inclusion complex and self-microemulsifying drug delivery system for photostability and enhanced oral bioavailability of methotrexate: novel technique. Drug Dev Ind Pharm 2013; 39(6): 918-27.
[http://dx.doi.org/10.3109/03639045.2012.718785] [PMID: 22998295]

[70]   Yan YD, Marasini N, Choi YK, *et al.* Effect of dose and dosage interval on the oral bioavailability of docetaxel in combination with a curcumin self-emulsifying drug delivery system (SEDDS). Eur J Drug Metab Pharmacokinet 2012; 37(3): 217-24.
[http://dx.doi.org/10.1007/s13318-011-0078-1] [PMID: 22201019]

[71]   He S, Cui Z, Mei D, *et al.* A cremophor-free self-microemulsified delivery system for intravenous injection of teniposide: evaluation *in vitro* and *in vivo*. AAPS PharmSciTech 2012; 13(3): 846-52.
[http://dx.doi.org/10.1208/s12249-012-9809-0] [PMID: 22644709]

[72]   Zhang L, Zhu W, Yang C, *et al.* A novel folate-modified self-microemulsifying drug delivery system of curcumin for colon targeting. Int J Nanomedicine 2012; 7: 151-62.
[PMID: 22275831]

[73]   Wu Z, Guo D, Deng L, Zhang Y, Yang Q, Chen J. Preparation and evaluation of a self-emulsifying drug delivery system of etoposide-phospholipid complex. Drug Dev Ind Pharm 2011; 37(1): 103-12.
[http://dx.doi.org/10.3109/03639045.2010.495752] [PMID: 21073324]

[74]   Wu X, Xu J, Huang X, Wen C. Self-microemulsifying drug delivery system improves curcumin dissolution and bioavailability. Drug Dev Ind Pharm 2011; 37(1): 15-23.
[http://dx.doi.org/10.3109/03639045.2010.489560] [PMID: 20738181]

[75]   Lo JT, Chen BH, Lee TM, Han J, Li JL. Self-emulsifying O/W formulations of paclitaxel prepared from mixed nonionic surfactants. J Pharm Sci 2010; 99(5): 2320-32.
[http://dx.doi.org/10.1002/jps.21993] [PMID: 19894274]

[76]   Lu JL, Wang JC, Zhao SX, *et al.* Self-microemulsifying drug delivery system (SMEDDS) improves anticancer effect of oral 9-nitrocamptothecin on human cancer xenografts in nude mice. Eur J Pharm Biopharm 2008; 69(3): 899-907.
[http://dx.doi.org/10.1016/j.ejpb.2008.02.023] [PMID: 18434109]

[77]   Quan DQ, Xu GX, Wu XG. Studies on preparation and absolute bioavailability of a self-emulsifying system containing puerarin. Chem Pharm Bull (Tokyo) 2007; 55(5): 800-3.
[http://dx.doi.org/10.1248/cpb.55.800] [PMID: 17473473]

[78]   Cui S, Zhao C, Chen D, He Z. Self-microemulsifying drug delivery systems (SMEDDS) for improving *in vitro* dissolution and oral absorption of Pueraria lobata isoflavone. Drug Dev Ind Pharm 2005; 31(4-5): 349-56.
[http://dx.doi.org/10.1081/DDC-54309] [PMID: 16093200]

[79]   Chae GS, Lee JS, Kim SH, *et al.* Enhancement of the stability of BCNU using self-emulsifying drug delivery systems (SEDDS) and *in vitro* antitumor activity of self-emulsified BCNU-loaded PLGA wafer. Int J Pharm 2005; 301(1-2): 6-14.
[http://dx.doi.org/10.1016/j.ijpharm.2005.03.034] [PMID: 16024190]

[80]   Taha EI, Samy AM, Kassem AA, Khan MA. Response surface methodology for the development of self-nanoemulsified drug delivery system (SNEDDS) of all-trans-retinol acetate. Pharm Dev Technol 2005; 10(3): 363-70.
[http://dx.doi.org/10.1081/PDT-65675] [PMID: 16176016]

[81]   Prajapati BG, Patel MM. Conventional and alternative pharmaceutical methods to improve oral bioavailability of lipophilic drugs. Asian J Pharm 2007; 1: 1-8.

[82]   Tang B, Cheng G, Gu JC, Xu CH. Development of solid self-emulsifying drug delivery systems: preparation techniques and dosage forms. Drug Discov Today 2008; 13(13-14): 606-12.
[http://dx.doi.org/10.1016/j.drudis.2008.04.006] [PMID: 18598917]

[83]   Almeida SRD, Tippavajhala VK. A Rundown through various methods used in the formulation of solid self-emulsifying drug delivery systems (S-SEDDS). AAPS PharmSciTech 2019; 20(8): 323.
[http://dx.doi.org/10.1208/s12249-019-1550-5]

[84]   Ameeduzzafar El-Bagory I, Alruwaili NK, Elkomy MH, *et al.* Development of novel dapagliflozin loaded solid self-nanoemulsifying oral delivery system: Physiochemical characterization and *in vivo* antidiabetic activity. J Drug Deliv Sci Technol 2019; 54: 101279.
[http://dx.doi.org/10.1016/j.jddst.2019.101279]

[85]   Abdalla A, Mäder K. Preparation and characterization of a self-emulsifying pellet formulation. Eur J Pharm Biopharm 2007; 66(2): 220-6.
[http://dx.doi.org/10.1016/j.ejpb.2006.11.015] [PMID: 17196807]

[86]   Gupta S, Kesarla R, Omri A. Formulation strategies to improve the bioavailability of poorly absorbed drugs with special emphasis on self-emulsifying systems. ISRN Pharm 2013; 2013: 848043.
[http://dx.doi.org/10.1155/2013/848043] [PMID: 24459591]

[87]   Ito Y, Kusawake T, Ishida M, Tawa R, Shibata N, Takada K. Oral solid gentamicin preparation using emulsifier and adsorbent. J Control Release 2005; 105(1-2): 23-31.
[http://dx.doi.org/10.1016/j.jconrel.2005.03.017] [PMID: 15908031]

[88]   Balakrishnan P, Lee BJ, Oh DH, *et al.* Enhanced oral bioavailability of dexibuprofen by a novel solid self-emulsifying drug delivery system (SEDDS). Eur J Pharm Biopharm 2009; 72(3): 539-45.
[http://dx.doi.org/10.1016/j.ejpb.2009.03.001] [PMID: 19298857]

[89]   El-Badry M, Fathy M. Enhancement of the dissolution and permeation rates of meloxicam by formation of its freeze-dried solid dispersions in polyvinylpyrrolidone K-30. Drug Dev Ind Pharm 2006; 32(2): 141-50.
[http://dx.doi.org/10.1080/03639040500465983] [PMID: 16537195]

[90]   Nazzal S, Smalyukh II, Lavrentovich OD, Khan MA. Preparation and *in vitro* characterization of a eutectic based semisolid self-nanoemulsified drug delivery system (SNEDDS) of ubiquinone: mechanism and progress of emulsion formation. Int J Pharm 2002; 235(1-2): 247-65.
[http://dx.doi.org/10.1016/S0378-5173(02)00003-0] [PMID: 11879759]

[91]   Pouton CW. Formulation of poorly water-soluble drugs for oral administration: physicochemical and physiological issues and the lipid formulation classification system. Eur J Pharm Sci 2006; 29(3-4): 278-87.
[http://dx.doi.org/10.1016/j.ejps.2006.04.016] [PMID: 16815001]

[92]   Soottitantawat A, Yoshii H, Furuta T, Ohkawara M, Linko P. Microencapsulation by spray drying: influence of emulsion size on the retention of volatile compounds. J Food Sci 2003; 68(7): 2256-62.
[http://dx.doi.org/10.1111/j.1365-2621.2003.tb05756.x]

[93]   Patil P, Joshi P, Paradkar A. Effect of formulation variables on preparation and evaluation of gelled self-emulsifying drug delivery system (SEDDS) of ketoprofen. AAPS PharmSciTech 2004; 5(3): e42.
[http://dx.doi.org/10.1208/pt050342] [PMID: 15760075]

[94]   Ahmad J, Mir SR, Kohli K, *et al.* Solid-nanoemulsion preconcentrate for oral delivery of paclitaxel: formulation design, biodistribution, and γ scintigraphy imaging. Biomed Res Int 2014; 2014: 984756.
[http://dx.doi.org/10.1155/2014/984756]

[95]   Itoh K, Tozuka Y, Oguchi T, Yamamoto K. Improvement of physicochemical properties of N-4472 part I formulation design by using self-microemulsifying system. Int J Pharm 2002; 238(1-2): 153-60.
[http://dx.doi.org/10.1016/S0378-5173(02)00085-6] [PMID: 11996819]

[96]   Gao P, Rush BD, Pfund WP, *et al.* Development of a supersaturable SEDDS (S-SEDDS) formulation of paclitaxel with improved oral bioavailability. J Pharm Sci 2003; 92(12): 2386-98.
[http://dx.doi.org/10.1002/jps.10511] [PMID: 14603484]

[97]   Serajuddin ATM, Sheen PC, Mufson D, Bernstein DF, Augustine MA. Effect of vehicle

amphiphilicity on the dissolution and bioavailability of a poorly water-soluble drug from solid dispersions. J Pharm Sci 1988; 77(5): 414-7.
[http://dx.doi.org/10.1002/jps.2600770512] [PMID: 3411464]

[98]   Sethia S, Squillante E. Solid dispersions: revival with greater possibilities and applications in oral drug delivery. Crit Rev Ther Drug Carrier Syst 2003; 20(2-3): 215-47.
[http://dx.doi.org/10.1615/CritRevTherDrugCarrierSyst.v20.i23.40] [PMID: 14584524]

CHAPTER 5

Targeting Approaches for the Diagnosis and Treatment of Cancer

Shivani Saraf[1], Ankita Tiwari[1], Amit Verma[1], Pritish K. Panda[1], Sarjana Raikwar[1], Ankit Jain[2], Rupal Dubey[3] and Sanjay K. Jain[1,*]

[1] Pharmaceutics Research Projects Laboratory, Department of Pharmaceutical Sciences, Dr. Hari Singh Gour Vishwavidyalaya, Sagar (M.P.) 470 003, India

[2] Institute of Pharmaceutical Research, GLA University, NH-2, Mathura-Delhi Road, Mathura (U.P.) 281 406, India

[3] School of Pharmacy and Research, People's University, Bhopal (M.P.) 462037, India

Abstract: Cancer is a multi-factorial disease that necessitates a multi-modality therapeutic approach to accomplish a favorable outcome. Recently, theranostic based systems have been introduced for the diagnosis coupled cancer therapy. The development of targeted novel drug/gene delivery approaches for safe and efficacious treatment of cancer is an emerging arena that includes liposomes, nanoparticles, nanoemulsion, gene therapy, immunosuppressant therapy, herbal bioactive loaded nanocarriers and stimuli sensitive systems (pH, temperature, ultrasound, redox potential, hypoxia and magnetic). Advancements in molecular biology have rendered a wide range of targeting moieties (ligands) and a meticulous understanding of the cancer biology is under extensive exploration for the selection of appropriate targets for cancer treatment. The outcomes of various clinical studies of nanocarriers depict an improvement in the anticancer efficacy and reduction in side effects. This chapter is an assemblage of advances in the novel targeting approaches that enable the cancer prevention, prediction, diagnosis and treatment.

Keywords: Cancer, Diagnosis, Liposomes, Nanocarriers, Nanoparticles.

INTRODUCTION

Tumor growth is a dynamic and complex process. Several factors such as complex angiogenesis, suppression of apoptosis, uncontrolled proliferation, escape from growth suppressor, increased invasion and metastasis, altered metabolism and evaded immune destruction may be involved in tumor growth and

[*] Corresponding author Sanjay K. Jain: Pharmaceutics Research Projects Laboratory, Department of Pharmaceutical Sciences, Dr. Hari Singh Gour Vishwavidyalaya, Sagar (M.P.) 470 003, India; Tel: +91-7582- 225782; E-mail: drskjainin@gmail.com

Atta-ur-Rahman and M. Iqbal Choudhary (Eds.)

dissemination [1, 2]. The tumor microenvironment (TME) consists of different cellular and non-cellular elements. The TME contains various non-malignant cells such as immune cells, bone marrow derived cells, inflammatory cells, extracellular matrix and tumor vasculature cells like cancer associated fibroblasts, endothelial cells and pericytes [3]. The stromal cells are recruited and stimulated by cancer cells. Stromal cells activate the biological signals and enhance the growth of fibroblasts which synthesize the chemokines, growth factors and adhesion molecules. The tumor stroma plays an important role in tumor metastasis and increases the capability to invade another cell. The cancerous cells are hypoxic in nature. Diffusion-limited hypoxia is caused due to restricted tumor vasculature since the tumor cells are distant from closest capillary as compared to the healthy cells (>100 μm) [4]. Due to the variation in oxygen delivery in blood vessels of tumor cells and oxygen consumption by cancer cells, there is a variation in their distance from blood vessels at which hypoxia occurs. Hypoxic condition in cancer cells causes stimulation of genes (hypoxia inducible factors 1 mediated) that are linked with angiogenesis process and cell survival. Such gene expressions may cause enhanced cell proliferation with modulated biochemical pathways which may resist the drug delivery [5]. Hypoxic areas of tumor cells have a reduced nutrient supply like glucose and amino acids. This is since cancer cells frequently utilize glycolysis to produce lactate in order to attain energy needed for cell survival and proliferation instead of oxidative metabolism, which efficiently leads to the generation of CO_2 and carbonic acid. Reduced metabolism and clearance of these acidic components cause low interstitial pH, which is another feature of tumors [6, 7]. Nanotechnology has been the area of interest over the last decade for developing precise carrier as it offers numerous benefits to overcome the limitations of conventional drug delivery system [8, 9]. It is a very promising platform for the treatment and diagnosis of cancer because it enters into the cells at molecular level. The nanotechnology is divided into different types like passive targeting, active targeting and stimuli responsive targeting. In case of passive targeting, the nanoparticles are preferentially retained into the tumor due to enhanced permeability and retention effect whereas in active targeting, the drug is preferentially delivered to the site of action [10]. Nanoparticles can be designed through various modifications such as changing their size, shape, chemical and physical properties, and so forth, to program them for targeting the desired cells. The nanocarriers are anchored with some ligands or antibodies for active targeting of drug. The target moiety facilitates the recognition of nanocarriers either by ligand receptor interaction or antibody-antigen recognition [11]. Nanocarriers have three basic components (i) chemotherapeutic agents (ii) targeting agents (ligand or antibody) and (iii) carriers (liposomes, nanoparticles, niosomes, dendrimers, *etc.*) [12 - 14]. Nanocarriers are usually made up of natural and synthetic polymers and lipids [15]. Accelerated clearance of nanocarriers from blood by reticulo-endothelial system uptake is the major drawback of novel drug delivery. Various approaches have been investigated to avoid the RES uptake and prolong the retention of nanocarriers in blood. The surface of nanocarriers is coated with hydrophilic polymers like polyethylene glycol (PEG), poloxamers, polysaccharides and poloxamines to avoid the elimination of carriers from opsonization. This phenomenon is known as "cloud" effect [16, 17]. The TME displays some unique features which can be used for active targeting of drug to the cancer cells. Cancer cells overexpress some receptors which can be utilized for active drug targeting. The ligands can be conjugated with nanocarriers which selectively bind to the receptor on tumor cells and internalized by receptor mediate endocytosis. Numerous studies are carried out to investigate interaction between ligand and receptor utilized for clinical use [18]. Further, stimuli sensitive nanocarriers came forth with recent advancements in nanotechnology. Several stimuli sensitive drug delivery systems have been used for the treatment of cancer like pH sensitive, temperature sensitive, photo sensitive, magnetic field responsive and hypoxia responsive drug delivery systems. They are made by stimuli responsive materials which change their properties in response to variations in the environment. They selectively release the drug in the presence of external or internal stimuli [19, 20]. The emerging growth of nanotechnology provides the opportunity to develop the multifunction delivery systems that allow the simultaneous detection, diagnosis, and treatment of tumor [21]. The theranostic system containing both diagnostic agent and drug in a single carrier can monitor the localization of drug at a specific site, visualize their biodistribution and assess therapeutic efficacy [22]. Ideal theranostic systems should: (i) localize into the cancer cells, (ii) visualize the biochemical and morphological changes of tumor cells, (iii) selectively deliver the drug to the target site without affecting the normal cells and (iv) be safe and biodegradable [23, 24].

DIAGNOSIS TECHNOLOGY

"Theranostics" is a new pharmaceutical strategy merging both diagnosis and treatment in a single delivery system. The theranostic nano-carrier contains therapeutic agents and diagnostic entities in a single system like liposomes or nanoparticles which monitor the treatment efficiency by proper imaging of disease and beneficial for more precise treatment of various complex diseases (Fig. **1**). The field of theranostic is uprising after the development of nanotechnology based carriers like nanoparticles, liposomes, dendrimers, micelles, and carbon nanotubes. It is one of the most potential approaches for targeting the cancer and providing the individualized treatment for cancer patients [25 - 27].

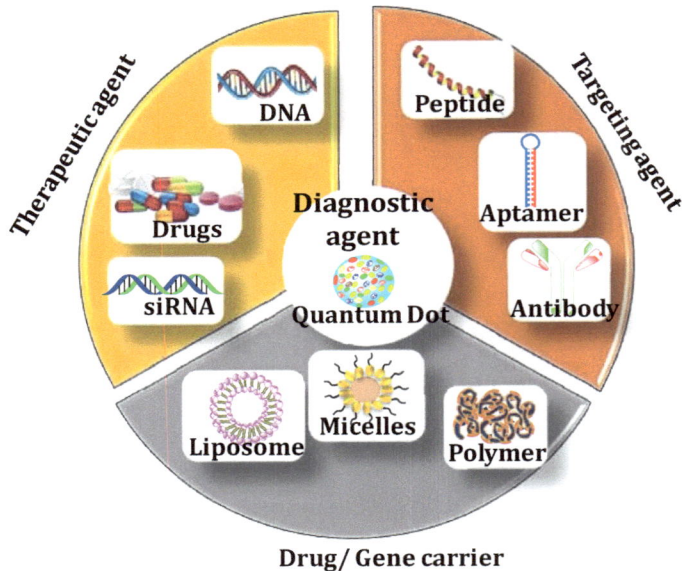

Fig. (1). Theranostic approaches for diagnosis and treatment of disease.

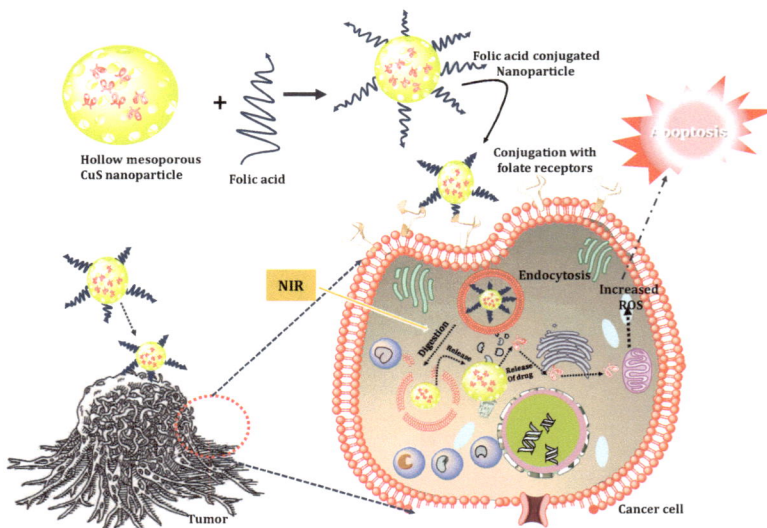

Fig. (2). Transferrin (Tf) conjugated hollow mesoporous CuS nanoparticles (HMCuS NPs) for targeted delivery of artesunate.

Personalized treatment for cancer using the combinatorial treatment is currently the most popular approach. A new approach namely diffusion molecular retention has been introduced for cancer targeting. The hollow mesoporous CuS nanoparticles (HMCuS NPs) modified with transferrin (Tf) were formulated and administered by a peritumoral (PT) injection (Fig. **2**). Iron-dependent artesunate, a cytotoxic drug was loaded into the nanoparticles which diffused through the interstitium and improved the retention in tumor site. The Tf-HMCuS NPs with strong near-infrared (NIR) absorption and photothermal conversion have been used in chemophototherapy. The Tf-mediated endocytosis was involved in uptake by MCF-7 cells and efficiently converted NIR light into heat for photothermal therapy which further generated the reactive oxygen species (ROS) for photodynamic therapy. The *in vivo* results demonstrated 74.8% tumor inhibition rate [28].

The polyarabic acid coated magnetic nanoparticles (PA-MNPs) containing the doxorubicin were prepared for the treatment of breast cancer. The coated nanoparticles improved the imaging, biocompatibility and therapeutic character. The polyarabic acid coating enhanced the penetration of nanoparticles into the cell membranes of breast cancer cells. The *in vivo* study was performed in mouse model of breast cancer. The outcomes of *in vivo* study revealed that the tumor growth was suppressed by PA-MNPs. The *in vivo* contrasting properties of PA-MNPs were compared with commercial gadolinium-based contrasting agents. The PA-MNPs possessed excellent contrasting power due to ferrous magnetic core and improved the imaging of cancer. The PA-MNPs were potential theranostic system for the treatment of cancers [29]. Graphene quantum dot (GQD)-based theranostic system modified with Herceptin (HER) and β-cyclodextrin (β-CD) was developed for the delivery of doxorubicin to breast cancer (Fig. **3**). The HER was used as a targeting ligand for HER2-overexpressed in breast cancer which improved the intracellular accumulation of doxorubicin in tumor cells.

β-CD (β-cyclodextrin) improved the loading efficiency of hydrophobic drug by providing the site to load *via* "host–guest" chemistry. The blue-color emission of the GQDs provided an effective diagnosis of tumor. The nanocarrier selectively degraded in tumor acidic environment and gradually released the doxorubicin to suppress the proliferation of tumor cells. The theranostic nanocarrier provided better diagnosis and treatment for HER2-overexpressed breast cancer [30]. Some theranostic based novel drug delivery systems are reported in Table **1**.

Table 1. Theranostic novel drug delivery systems.

System	Ligand	Chemotherapeutic Agent	Model Imaging Agent	Type of Cancer	Refs.
Nanoparticles	Hyaluronic acid (HA)	Doxorubicin	NIR fluorescent imaging (NIR dye)	Ovarian cancer	[31]

(Table 1) cont.....

System	Ligand	Chemotherapeutic Agent	Model Imaging Agent	Type of Cancer	Refs.
Micelles of D-α-tocopheryl polyethylene glycol 1000 succinate (TPGS)	Transferring	Docetaxel	Ultra bright gold clusters (AuNC)	Breast cancer	[32]
Prodrug micelles	Hyaluronic acid	Doxorubicin	AIE fluorogentetraphenylene (TPE); (TPE units with typical AIE characteristics)	Breast cancer	[33]
Nanoparticles (NPs)	Folic acid		Mn: ZnS quantum dots	Breast cancer	[34]
Nanoparticles	Folic acid	Cytotoxic peptide (CT20p)	Near infrared fluorescent dye	Prostate cancer	[35]
Nanoemulsions	Folate	Docetaxel (DTX)	NMI-500	Ovarian cancer	[36]
Magnetic iron oxide nanoparticles (IONPs)	Recombinant amino terminal fragment (ATF) peptides	Doxorubicin	Near infrared dye	Pancreatic cancer	[37]

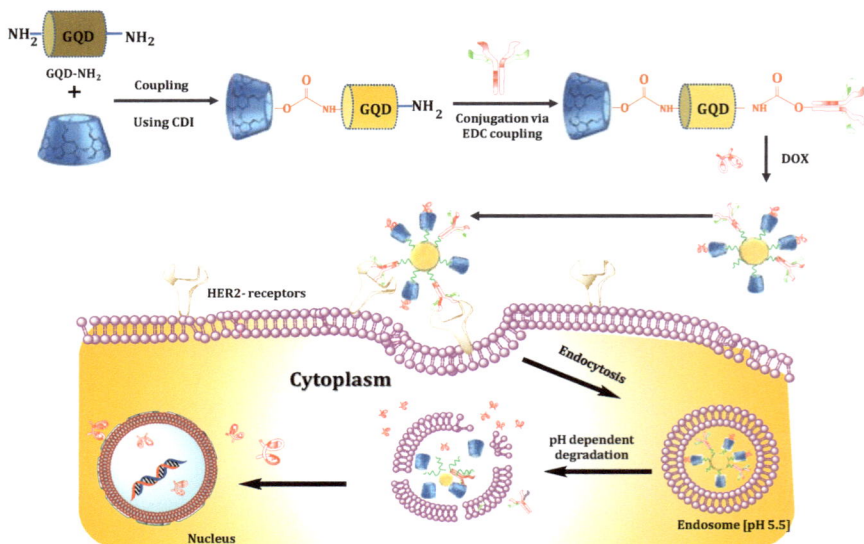

Fig. (3). Development of DOX-loaded HER labeled GQD based nanocarrier and its cellular uptake for active targeting of breast cancer.

RECENT APPROACHES FOR THE TREATMENT OF CANCER

Targeted Drug Delivery Carriers

Liposomes

Liposomes are bilayered structures made up of phospholipid and cholesterol. They can encapsulate both hydrophilic and hydrophobic drugs [38 - 40]. Combinatorial administration of Paclitaxel (PTX) and imatinib in liposomes would be an effective approach for the optimization of cancer therapy [41]. Surface modified liposomal preparation using distearoyl phosphatidyl ethanolamine-polyethylene glycol (2000)-folic acid (DSPE-PEG$_{2000}$-FA) lipid conjugate was developed by combining the above drugs for targeting folate receptor. Lyophilized preparation depicted stability for a span of 2 months in terms of drug loading and size. Folic acid-targeted liposomes exhibited a greater suppression on MCF-7 cell viability in comparison to the free PTX and non-targeted liposomes. In prostate cancer cell line *i.e.,* PC-3 cells, viability curtailment was more in the case of liposomes entrapping both drugs relative to the non-targeted liposomal preparation. VEGF gene expression was observed to decrease in MCF7 and PC-3 cells, with targeted liposomes which are displaying better activity as compared to non-targeted liposomes [42]. Gadolinium (Gd) entrapped liposomes modified with aptamer were developed for efficient diagnosis of cancer using magnetic resonance imaging (MRI). GBI-10$_m$ (modified form of GBI-10 aptamer) was employed for the fabrication of targeted liposomes (G$_m$Ls). Liposomes with GBI-10 aptamer (GLs) and without aptamer (untargeted) were taken as controls. It was depicted that G$_m$Ls were remarkably more in cytoplasm as compared to GLs, and G$_m$Ls and GLs were more compared to untargeted liposomes. In flow cytometry, the fluorescence intensity of G$_m$Ls was raised by two folds than the intensity of GLs and thrice more than that of non-targeted liposomes. Thus, the G$_m$Ls proved their potential as MRI contrast agent at a temperature of 37°C for the recognition of cancer cells with overexpressed tenascin-C (protein) [43]. Entrapment of Polyethylenimine/oligonucleotides (ODN) in liposomes is desirable for the *in vivo* administration of nucleic acid based moieties. Nevertheless, toxicity caused by polyethylenimine limits its clinical applicability. In order to overcome this limitation, polyplexes encapsulated in liposomes were prepared by replacing polyethylenimine with low molecular weight chitosan. The cationic polyplexes were loaded into negatively charged liposomes with the help of membrane extrusion. Folate-conjugated phospholipid was used for the development of folate-targeted liposomes entrapping low molecular weight chitosan (LMWC)/oligonucleotide (ODN) polyplexes [LS (CO)]. The LS (CO) and folate targeted liposomes encapsulating

LS (CO) [FLS (CO)] depicted a mean diameter ~130 nm and neutral zeta potential and stayed stable for a period of one week in 0.15-M NaCl at 25°C. FLS (CO) revealed greater cellular uptake compared to LS (CO) in B16F10 murine melanoma cells. Moreover, LS (CO) demonstrated lower toxicity than polyethylenimine/oligonucleotides entrapped in liposomes, depicting a biocompatible novel carrier system of oligonucleotides [44]. Combinatorial delivery of drugs by entrapping them in liposomes has grabbed the attention of scientists since maximum synergistic action of entrapped drugs is attained. Many researchers have asserted that the combined regimen of mitoxantrone (MTO) and prednisolone (PLP) depicts a synergistic anticancer effect. Low molecular weight heparin-sodium deoxy cholate conjugate -modified liposomes (PLP-MTO-HM) were developed using liposome fusion method. The co-localization of DiD-C--HM dyes took place in tumor cells, whereas, no co-localization could be observed in co-administered DiD-HM and C6-CM till 24 h. In CT26 and B16F10 mouse models, the developed liposomes depicted remarkably greater tumor suppression in comparison to the co-administration of MTO-HM and PLP-CM. The outcomes evidenced that the developed system displayed better anticancer effect in comparison to co-administration therapy because of the synergistic effect [45]. In majority of cancers, mutation of p53 (tumor suppressor gene) takes place which leads to the aberrance in the p53 pathway. A liposomal nanocomplex SGT-53 employing an anti-transferrin receptor single-chain antibody fragment as a targeting ligand was developed for systemic targeting of p53 gene. It depicted good targeting potential in patients of advanced solid tumors in phase 1. An increased anticancer potential was noted in preclinical analysis when SGT-53 and docetaxel were administered in a combination. Therefore, this trial was attempted in 14 advanced cancer patients for safety and efficacy assessment of the combination. The outcomes disclosed that SGT-53 (3.6 mg DNA/infusion) and docetaxel (75 mg/m^2/infusion) when taken in a combination were well tolerated. Furthermore, its activity was evaluated in 12 patients. Among them, three patients attained response evaluation criteria in solid tumor (RECIST)-verified partial responses with tumor suppression of -47%, -51%, and -79%. In two patients, a remarkable shrinkage (-25% and -16%) in tumor tissues was observed. The outcomes revealed that SGT-53 and docetaxel in combinatorial delivery could be testified for phase 2 clinical trials [46]. Gene therapy is an emerging field in cancer therapy but its applicability is restrained since systemic delivery of therapeutics cannot target multifocal cancer. A liposomal nanocomplex *i.e.* SGT-94 bearing a plasmid encoding RB94 was formulated for targeted systemic delivery to tumor. In the preclinical analysis, RB94 demonstrated remarkable tumor cytotoxicity but no signs of toxicity were seen in healthy cells. The intravenous delivery of SGT-94 for metastatic genitourinary cancer is currently in phase I - clinical trial. It showed minimum side effects and dose-limiting toxicity

(DLT). Moreover, it exhibited tumor- targeting of SGT-94 complex [47].

Nanoparticles

Nanoparticles are the most commonly used novel drug delivery system for the treatment of cancer [48]. PTX entrapped in lipid core nanoparticles (LDE) showed close resemblance with the chemical structure of low density lipoprotein (LDL) which decreased the toxicity in a significant manner. This PTX-LDE system was also tested (74 chemotherapy cycles) for its safety in the third-line treatment for ovarian cancer and no toxicity signs were noticed in any of the cycles [49]. The efficiency of drugs which target vascular endothelial growth factor (VEGF) pathway is restricted by raised hypoxia cells and hypoxia-inducible factor-1α (HIF1α). A combination of anti-angiogenic drugs with HIF1α inhibiting moieties could be a promising approach to countervail it. CRLX101 (nanoparticle-drug conjugate holding camptothecin) was assessed as a single agent and combined with bevacizumab in model of metastatic ovarian cancer in mice. Preclinically, CRLX101 is efficient as a monotherapy when delivered at maximal-tolerated doses. Moreover, low-dose CRLX101 with bevacizumab decreased bevacizumab-mediated HIF1α up-regulation and led to synergistic effect with minimum toxicity in mice. Parallelly, CRLX101 depicted 74% tumor inhibition in clinical trials phase II. The assessment revealed the efficiency of CRLCX101 alone or in combination with bevacizumab in the treatment of ovarian cancer. It can also be tested for application in other types of cancer which involve HIF1α in their pathogenesis as it can enhance the efficiency of anti-angiogenic agents [50]. Drug carrier systems which are based on surface-engineered magnetic nanoparticles have sought the attention of the researchers as these systems could be delivered to the target site and drug could be released due to change in pH, temperature, radiation, or even magnetic field. The reticulo-endothelial system quickly removes the particles from the blood thereby reducing their half-lives. Therefore, it is essential to coat them with suitable materials which could evade the macrophagic uptake and enhance their biocompatibility. Polymer namely poly (butylcyanoacrylate) was coated on magnetic nanoparticles and they were characterized for physical properties and as a system for magnetically controlled drug delivery. Various analyses like infrared spectroscopy, electrophoretic mobility, thermodynamics study, and X-ray affirmed an adequate polymer coating on the particles. Besides, assays on normal colon and breast cancer cell lines *i.e.* CCD-18 and MCF-10A, respectively and colon and breast cancer cell lines T-84 and MCF-7, respectively, evidenced that nanocomposites showed very less cytotoxicity in normal cell lines and significant cytotoxicity in tumor cell lines [51]. A novel delivery system was developed by the conjugation of methoxy-poly(ethylene glycol)-block-poly(6-O-methacryloyl-D-galacto- pyranose) (mPEG

-b-PMAGP) and doxorubicin (DOX) through an acid-labile carbamate linkage. The DOX cumulative release from the developed nanoparticles was observed to be 26.58% during 72 h at pH 7.4. It was remarkably slower as compared to the release at pH 6.5 (43.61%) and 5.0 (74.68%). It may be because of the carbamate link degradation amongst polymer and DOX in response to changes in pH. The mPEG-b-PMAGP-co-DOX nanoparticles containing galactose groups displayed higher cell uptake *via* asialoglycoprotein receptor-mediated endocytosis process in HepG2 cells as compared to the other tumor cells. It was evidenced from the *in vitro* cytotoxicity assay that the developed nanoparticles demonstrated greater anticancer activity against HepG2 cells in comparison to MCF-7 cells. The developed pH-responsive system could be used to target hepatoma [52]. Functional nucleic acids are extensively employed in cancer therapy as they get triggered by stimuli and effectively target the cancer cells. The major hurdles in nucleic acid based nanocarriers are high cost, poor bio-stability and complex development process. pH-responsive doxorubicin (Dox) nanoparticles were prepared for cancer targeting exploiting the benefit of rolling circle amplification (RCA) method, using which large amount of functional DNAs could be effectively collected. Moreover, Mg^{2+}, main electrolyte in body depicting better biocompatibility, can adequately condense the sequence of an RCA product and conserve its functions. *In vitro* drug release was conducted during a 72-h time duration at pH 7.4 and 5.0. At pH 7.4, magnesium-RCA Nanoclew maximally loaded doxorubicin (Mg-RNC1@Dox) released < 8% during the entire period and at pH 5.0, Mg-RNC1@Dox depicted a sustained release throughout the 72-h time; while a burst release was initially found for magnesium pyrophosphate-RCA Nanoclew (MgPPi-RNC1@Dox). The DNA nanoparticles were bio-stable rendering, them an ideal system for *in vivo* delivery. This would find many applications in the arena of biomedicine [53].

Nanoemulsion

Applications of nanoparticles in therapy are tremendously rising in the last few decades. Besides their drug targeting ability and bioavailability enhancement capability, nanoparticles can permit their detection using a wide range of imaging techniques. A nanoparticle system was designed to image directed therapy, and it was assessed in colon cancer in mice. The "theranostic" system is based on oil-in-water nanoemulsion and it holds Cy7 (fluorescent dye) for NIRF imaging, prednisolone acetate valerate for therapeutic applications and iron oxide nanocrystals for MRI. MRI and NIRF imaging of nanoemulsion modified with $\alpha_v\beta_3$-targeted RGD peptides depicted remarkable accumulation of the system in the cancer cells, whereas cancer growth profiles displayed a potent inhibitory effect in all animals treated with nanoemulsion as compared to the treatment with control nanoemulsion, the drug or saline [54]. Among all the cancers in women, 23% of the new cases and 13.7% of all deaths are accounted by breast cancer. Chemotherapy poses many undesirable effects on healthy cells, leading to multidrug resistance and raised toxicity to normal cells. With an aim to increase the anticancer potency of docetaxel (DTX), it was encapsulated in lipid particles (Folate-conjugated PEG-solid fat nanoemulsion) stabilized using soya phosphatidylcholine (PC) for targeting breast cancer. The IC_{50} of plain solid fat nanoemulsion, folate-conjugated PEG-solid fat nanoemulsion and docetaxel solution were observed to be 14.2, 64.9, and 28.8 and 14.2 μM/ml, respectively. The treatment of HeLa cells with folate-conjugated PEG-solid fat nanoemulsion showed fluorescence which depicted more cellular uptake of ligand-appended nanoemulsion as compared to plain solid fat nanoemulsion. It could be explored for target specific and non-immunogenic delivery of therapeutic agents for the treatment of various diseased conditions [55]. PTX is widely utilized for targeting breast, non-small cell lung, pancreatic cancer, *etc.* But its poor water solubility (<1 μg/mL) limits its application. In order to overcome this limitation, HA-modified PTX nanoemulsion (HPNs) was developed by ionic complexation of PTX nanoemulsion and HA to target non-small cell lung cancer. The *in vivo* anticancer efficiency of the nanoemulsion was evaluated by assessing the alterations in tumor volume and body weight in nude mice which were transplanted with CD44-overexpressing NCI-H460 xenografts followed by treatment with saline, Taxol®, PTX nanoemulsion (PNs), or HPNs (dose 25 mg/kg). Inhibition of tumor cell growth was greater in the PNs- and HPN-treated groups as compared to the Taxol® group. HPN treatment significantly suppressed tumor growth, probably due to the specific cancer -targeting affinity of HA ligand for CD44-overexpressed tumor cells. It is concluded that HPNs could be effectively employed for targeting non-small cell lung cancer overexpressing CD44 [56].

Hydrogel

Local chemotherapy is a potential treatment strategy for controlling the tumor growth [57]. The nanotechnology based systems are used for local chemotherapy [58]. Hydrogel is an effective treatment strategy for local chemotherapy. The hydrogels are biocompatible and biodegradable delivery system. The stimuli responsive gel systems like temperature sensitive, pH sensitive, electric fields responsive delivery systems are suitable carriers for local chemotherapy [59]. These implantable gel systems have swelling properties and show controlled drug release for the localized cancer treatment. The temperature responsive chitosan and β-glycerophosphate salt-based hydrogel incorporated with polyethylenimine modified super-paramagnetic graphene oxide were formulated for the effective management of cancer. The system improved the antitumor activity in presence of an alternating magnetic field (AMF) [60]. The *in situ* gel forming self-assembling peptide as a depot system was formulated for delivery of doxorubicin (DOX) and curcumin (CUR). *In vitro* release study demonstrated that DOX- *in situ* gel displayed the sustained release of DOX for 4 days and CUR- *in situ* gel prolonged the release of CUR for 20 days. DOX-*in situ* gel improved the cytotoxicity in comparison to free DOX. The CUR-*in situ* gels enhanced the apoptosis activity than free CUR. Therefore, the depot system was the potential carrier for sustained delivery of chemotherapeutic agents [61]. Silibinin is herbal agent which depicts the antitumor potential. The temperature sensitive hydogel was developed for the delivery of silibinin to tumor cells. The MTT assay, clonogenic assay, flow cytometry and Western blot technique were utilized to assess the antitumor potential of hydrogel. The formulation suppressed the cell proliferation, stimulated the cell arrest induced apoptosis and suppressed the oncogenic pathways (*i.e.* STAT3 and MEK/ERK) in B16-F10 cells [62].

Gene Therapy

Gene therapy is an emerging field which has huge potential for cancer drug targeting and it may be used alone or in combination with the available treatment approaches. It includes mainly gene transfer therapy, immunotherapy and oncolytic virotherapy. Gene transfer therapy is a newer approach in which the new genes are introduced into the tumour cells and they either slow down the growth of the cancerous cells or cause their death. In immunotherapy, viral particles and cells, which are modified genetically, are utilized to trigger the immune system and target various kinds of cancer. Oncolytic virotherapy comprises the viral elements which have the ability to replicate inside the tumour cells and cause their death. The viruses generally used are naturally oncolytic, or engineered from the original non-oncolytic viruses. They trigger the antitumor immune response by encoding immune-stimulatory cytokines in order to improve the oncolytic potency. The first oncolytic virus therapy was developed for the treatment of melanoma in the year 2015 and got approved by FDA [63, 64]. Presently, gene therapy is used to develop recombinant cancer vaccines. Generally, cancer cells are collected from the patients or from established cancer cell lines and are grown *in vitro*. Further, they are modified for the better recognition by immune system with the help of one or more genes. These genes may be the cytokine genes which produce pro-inflammatory immune stimulating molecules, or highly antigenic protein genes which are incorporated into a vaccine. These genes produce proteins which trigger the development of antitumor antibodies [65]. The first approved gene transfer study was done in 1989 at the National Institutes of Health (NIH). Many of the cancer including skin, colon, prostate, lung, gynecological, urological, neurological and gastrointestinal tumors as well as hematological malignancies have been targeted *via* gene therapy.

Aptamer Based System

Aptamers are single-stranded RNA or DNA oligonucleotides bearing relatively small molecular weight *i.e.* nearly one-tenth that of monoclonal antibodies and have a distinct ability to fold into unique three-dimensional structures. They have good binding capability for a variety of targets such as metal ions, small molecules, proteinous substances, viruses, bacteria and whole cells with high specificity and binding affinities similar to the antibodies. Currently, aptamers are the best suitable agents for the discovery of biomarkers as well as for the diagnostic and therapeutic applicability in cancer. Aptamers are small in size and have several advantages as compared to antibodies like low immunogenicity, high tissue penetration, rapid *in vitro* selection and cell-free chemical synthesis, *etc*. Aptamers are isolated and randomly selected from the oligonucleotide library. Then, the identified aptamers are synthesized, modified, optimized and utilized for cancer targeting [66]. Systematic evolution of ligands by exponential enrichment (SELEX) is a simple and common technique to detect the metastatic cells in cancer cell lines. It has four steps: incubation, partition, recovery, and amplification. An aptamer for colon cancer was developed with the help of SELEX where LoVo cells were used for positive selection and SW480 and HT-29 cells were used for negative selection. The aptamer, labelled with cyanine (Cy5, a fluorescent dye) was detected in lymphatic tissue (detection rate 73.9%) of metastatic colon cancer patients [67]. Duan *et al.* prepared an aptamer, DML-7, for prostate cancer (PCa) by using SELEX with DU145 and WPMY-1 cell lines for positive selection and counter selection, respectively. This aptamer was then verified for androgen receptor (AR)-negative (PC3) and AR-positive (LNCaP and 22Rv1). ARs play a crucial role in the progression of PCa but may suppress the metastasis. Clinical studies demonstrated that ARs are down-regulated in metastatic PCa. It was observed that DML-7 bound to PC-3 cells but not to LNCaP and 22Rv1 cells [68]. Chen *et al.* (2016) developed an aptamer for the management of hepatocellular carcinoma which demonstrated that it has high specificity to HCCLM9 cell line but did not bind to any other cell lines [69]. MMP-9 is over-expressed in many cancers and promotes metastasis by degrading the extracellular matrix thereby helping in cancer cell invasion It was successfully targeted by an RNA aptamer [70].

Aptamers for Easy and Early Detection of Cancer

Six advanced DNA aptamers having magnetic properties were prepared using carboxyl agar beads. It was developed by modified SELEX technique and used against lung cancer. These aptamers precisely helped in the detection of tumor cells in the serum of lung cancer patients [71]. Besides, an advanced aptamer based microfluidic system was designed for the diagnosis of circulating tumor cells (CTCs), which are commonly observed in minute concentrations and circulate irregularly. With the utilization of such particular aptamers, the system helps for quick detection in comparison to antibody-based diagnosis of ovarian cancer [72].

Clinical Trials of Cancer-Targeting Aptamers

AS1411 is a DNA oligonucleotide which was the first aptamer that entered in clinical trials for cancer treatment. It has strong affinity for nucleolin which is found to be overexpressed in the nuclei and surfaces of tumor cells; involved in growth, proliferation and survival of the cells. Once it binds to the nucleolin, it is internalized proficiently into the cell. It has the potential to inhibit the function of nucleolin in carcinogenic cells and exhibits more anti-proliferative activity in all type of cancers such as lung, cervical, prostate, breast, skin, blood and colon cancer. In phase I clinical trial, infusion of a dose of 40 mg/kg/day of AS1411 was delivered which inhibited nucleolin with minute toxic effects [73]. NOX-A12 is a 45-nt L-ribose-based RNA aptamer (trade name Spiegelmer) which has the ability to resist the nucleases enzyme [74]. Moreover, it has the capability to link with polyethylene glycol (40kDa) to improve its plasma half-life [75].

Antibody Based System

Antibody-based systems have become well-known over the last 15-20 years for cancer targeting. Recently, it has egressed as a potential strategy for the treatment of various cancer malignancies [76].

TMAs (Therapeutic Monoclonal Antibodies)

These are the most commonly used antibodies having the potential to overcome the side effects that are associated with cancer chemotherapy. Recently, these have been used in targeted drug delivery. The first TMA (Orthoclone OKT3®) was discovered and approved by the FDA in September 1992. Numerous TMAs have undergone for preclinical and clinical investigations. Currently, more than

12 TMAs are used in cancer therapy and about 40 TMAs got regulatory approval. For the successful preparation of TMAs, an expertise in technical capability is required for handling the genetically engineered chimeric or humanized antibodies. Various techniques have been investigated for increasing the blood TMA half-life and strengthening the immune action. More understanding in cancer cell biology and their targeting as well as the immune and non-immunological concepts carry forward the antibody based targeting systems. In IgFc glycosylation, it revealed that the antibody-dependent cellular cytotoxicity (ADCC) was affected when the fucose moieties bound to the CH_2 side of the heavy chain of the antibody. It was also reported that the engineered IgG antibodies which did not have fucosylated oligosaccharides enhance the ADCC activity both *in vitro* and *in vivo*. Moreover, a sound knowledge of various parameters is required for the selection of lead antibody, patient study groups and actual design of clinical trials which include the distribution of antigen in target versus normal tissues, pharmacokinetics study of antibody, efficiency in different models and the antibody uptake inside the cancerous tissue. The first TMA prepared for cancer therapy was Rituxin or Rituximab, which is a cell-surface glycosylated phosphor-protein. It is a chimeric antibody targeting CD20 used for the treatment of Non-Hodgkin's B-cell Lymphoma (NHL) [77, 78]. Ibritumomab was developed by conjugating the monoclonal antibody with the yttrium isotope and got approved in the year 2002 for the management of NHL and Rituxin-refractory lymphoma. It is a murine anti CD20 monoclonal antibody (MA). Besides, an immune radioisotope, situmomab-I131, was also approved in the year 2003 for the treatment of patients with CD20 positive Follicular Lymphoma (FL) [79, 80]. Mapatumumab is a humanized IgG1 antibody which targets TRAIL R1 antigen has been developed for the management of cervical cancer. Obinutuzumab was prepared by glycol-engineered in Chinese Hamster ovary (CHO) cells. It showed different activity than anti CD20 MA because Asp297 was glycosylated with CH_2 Fc region of the MA. Because of this modification, the ADCC activity was increased while the complement dependent cytotoxicity (CDC) activity was decreased. Further, point alterations were noticed in some variable region sequences by an epitope named GA-101 that resulted in increased binding affinity [81]. Ofatumumab, an IgG1 based anti-CD20 antibody, was investigated and got approval in the year 2009 by the FDA for the treatment of chronic lymphocytic leukemia (CLL). Veltuzumab is a type 1 humanized anti-CD20, IgG1 MA used for non-Hodgkin lymphoma (NHL) and CLL [82]. Ocrelizumab is also a Type 1 humanized anti-CD20, IgG1 antibody which has the tendency to bind to a similar epitope as that of Rituxin. Fc region of the antibody has been modified in order to improve its binding affinity for the FcγRIII that is useful in the management of leukemia [83]. Alemtuzumab is a fully-humanized IgG1 antibody approved in the year 2001 by FDA and it has the ability to target

CD52, and used for CLL. It induces apoptosis by promoting both ADCC and CDC [84]. Milatuzumab is also a type of humanized antibody which targets CD74 in B-cell leukemias [85].

Antibody Drug Conjugates (ADCs)

The development of ADCs requires two essential factors. The first factor includes drug potency. Previous studies reported that a fewer quantities of antibody was deposited due to slow mass transfer inside the solid tumors. This drawback can be overcome by using some of the potent drugs in ADCs like the uristatins and maytansinoids (microtubule inhibitors) and calicheamycin or duocarmycin analogs (DNA-damaging agents), *etc*. The second factor is to synthesize suitable linker molecules required for the coupling of drugs to the antibody [86, 87]. To date, a few ADCs have got FDA approvals for cancer therapy and considered for clinical use. Trastuzumab emtansine (T-DM1) is comprised of antibody Trastuzumab (Herceptin) which targets the HER-2 cell surface protein used for the treatment of breast cancer [88]. Gemtuzumab ozogamicin (Mylotag) is a recombinant conjugate, humanized IgG4 MA developed to target CD33. The antibody was prepared for linking to calicheamycin and got approval in the year 2000 by FDA, for the management of acute myelogenous leukemia [89]. Brentuximab vedotin (Adcetris) constitutes of a chimeric antibody intended to target CD30 which was found to be overexpressed on T or B-cell lymphomas. It is used as a tumor marker in some of the carcinogenic conditions in lymphomas and certain embryonal carcinomas [90]. Inotuzumab ozogamicin (CMC-544) contains IgG4 MA, that was developed to target the CD22 antigen which are located on mature B cells [91]. Lorvotuzumab mertansine (IMGN901) is a humanized MA which targets CD56 and generally expressed on NK cells, few T-cells and in Multiple Myeloma [92]. Recently, many of the ADCs have been developed and are in different stages of preclinical and clinical trials.

Stimuli Sensitive Drug Delivery Systems

Stimuli sensitive drug delivery systems (DDS) are defined as the systems which respond to the stimuli like pH, temperature, magnetic field and light for delivering bioactive(s) to target site. Various types of stimulus-responsive DDS have been effectively designed using nanotechnology and efficacy of these systems was confirmed by preclinical animal experiments [93 - 100]. Nanocarriers based stimuli-responsive drug delivery is used to attain cancer specific targeting with high therapeutic effects and low side effects. The characteristics of tumor microenvironment like higher temperature, lower pH and overexpressed proteolytic enzymes are the key biomarkers for the preparation of stimuli sensitive

DDS [101 - 103]. The stimuli sensitive nanocarriers have been introduced in the field of cancer therapeutics. These systems offer many advantages like improved pharmacokinetic parameters, better retention, increased cell uptake and drug release selectively in the diseased area in response to internal or external stimuli (*e.g.,* cancer) [93, 104 - 106]. The main objective of an ideal carrier system is to accomplish the concentration of drug within a desirable therapeutic range after administration, and localize the medicament to preferred site while reducing its amount in non-target sites [107]. Hu *et al.* developed a novel pluronicF127/ graphene nanohybrid (GN) pH responsive drug delivery system. The nanohybrid displayed 56% and 25% of drug release at pH 5 and 9, respectively in 90 h. The amount of DOX release at acidic pH was higher than that of neutral and basic pH. PF127/GN loaded DOX (PF127/GN/DOX) showed significant cytotoxicity to the MCF-7 as compared to PF127/GN nanohybrid [108]. Stimuli sensitive DDS retain their structural integrity throughout circulation and trigger the drug release in response to particular stimuli at the target site. These systems are fabricated to endure faster changes within the tumor microenvironment like disruption, aggregation of system leading to triggered drug release [109 - 112]. Various stimuli-sensitive nanocarriers have been discussed below.

pH Sensitive Drug Delivery Systems

The pH responsive systems respond to the change in the pH of surrounding area in case of specific disease like cancer [113 - 116]. Crayton *et al.* developed a pH-titratable super paramagnetic Fe_2O_3 nanoparticles for improving the accumulation of nanoparticles in acidic microenvironment of tumor [117]. They developed pH-responsive Fe_2O_3 nanoparticles using glycol chitosan (GC). The GC was conjugated on the surface of super paramagnetic iron oxide nanoparticles (SPIO) in order to produce a T2 (transverse relaxation time) weighted magnetic resonance contrast agent that responds to variations in pH. The formulation showed pH dependent potent cellular association as compared to simple nanoparticles. Zhou *et al.* (2014) reported the targeted and controlled delivery of DOX by synthesizing a graphene oxide (GO) nanosystem functionalized with charge reversal polyelectrolyte and integrin $\alpha_v\beta_3$mono antibody. The drug release study demonstrated that the nanocarriers have high efficiency along with effective drug release at acidic pH. They used anionic carboxylate functional polyelectrolyte (charge-reversal polyelectrolyte), poly(allylamine hydrochloride)-citraconic anhydride (PAH-Cit), which can be easily converted into cationic poly allylamine by amide hydrolysis in response to slightly acidic condition and release the DOX into target tumor cells [118]. Feng *et al.* (2014) prepared a pH-sensitive nanoscale graphene oxide (NGO) by coating the surface of NGO with two types of polymers, polyethylene glycol (PEG) and poly allylamine hydrochloride. The system was further modified with 2,3 dimethylmaleic anhydride (DA) in order to impart pH dependent charge reversibility. The dual sensitive NGO PEG DA/DOX complex showed higher cellular uptake under the acidic pH of tumor, and augmented the release of DOX within the lysosomal pH. The combination of phototherapy and chemotherapy by NGO PEG DA/DOX complex provided an additive effect and overcame the drug resistance [119]. Lue *et al.* (2014) developed an innovative HCO_3^- bearing nanocarrier having pH-sensitive characteristics, which can produce carbon dioxide gas and facilitate the drug release. The reaction between HCO_3^- and acid produces carbonic acid, which is further, degraded to form CO_2 gas and H_2O molecules. Consequently, HCO_3^- bearing nanoparticles triggered the release of drug selectively in the acidic pH [120]. Ke *et al.* (2011) prepared PLGA hollow microspheres (HM) that could deliver anticancer drugs (DOX) into cancer cells leading to the burst release of drug in acidic microenvironment. The hydrogen ion reacts with $NaHCO_3$ to form CO_2 bubbles, which leads to the release of DOX at acidic pH of tumor [121].

Temperature Sensitive Drug Delivery Systems

Temperature is the most important stimulus in stimuli sensitive DDS. There are two types of thermo responsive polymers *i.e.* lower critical solution temperature type polymers and upper critical solution temperature (UCST) type polymers. The lower critical solution temperature type of polymer dissolves in water at temperature lower than lower critical solution temperature (LCST) but they are insoluble at temperatures above LCST, *e.g.*, Poly (N-isopropylacrylamide) (PNIPAM) [122 - 124], N,N-diethylacrylamide (DEAM) [125], while UCST types of polymer become soluble upon heating *e.g.*, combination of acrylamide (AAM) and acrylic acid (AAc) [126]. Staruch *et al.* (2015) developed thermo-sensitive liposomes in which hyperthermia mediated drug release was triggered by magnetic resonance high intensity focussed ultrasound (MR HIFU) and antitumor effect was determined in rabbit VX2 tumors. The rabbit was treated with a single dose of thermosensitive liposomal DOX infusion with MR HIFU. The tumor growth was reduced rapidly due to faster release of DOX at higher temperature [127]. A temperature sensitive liposomal system was developed using a temperature sensitive lysolipid to improve the efficacy for chemotherapy [128, 129]. This formulation was studied in the clinical trials (Phase III) for the management of hepatocellular carcinoma and also in phase II clinical trials for breast cancer and metastatic colorectal cancer.

Magnetic Sensitive Drug Delivery Systems

Magnetic field is another essential stimuli, non-invasive energy source which plays a crucial role in sustained release of drugs from magnetic field responsive nanocarriers [130]. The magnetic field is applied either locally to increase the deposition of drug in the tumor, or by alternating the magnetic field to induce tumor heating to achieve better anticancer efficacy. Magnetic stimuli facilitate the delivery of anti-cancerous drug to target sites and maintain its concentration in blood up to its complete absorption [111]. Zhu *et al.* (2012) prepared magnetized liposomes using magnetites, such as Fe_3O_4 or glutamic acid-chelated Fe_2O_3 (γ-Fe_2O_3) that is less than 10 nm in size. They co-loaded methotrexate and γ-Fe_2O_3 inside the core (aqueous) of liposomes. The *in vivo* study in mouse model demonstrated that the magnetic carrier considerably enhanced the methotrexate accumulation by more than 5 folds in the target tissue when exposed to MF as compared to the same formulation without an external magnetic stimulus [131].

Redox Sensitive Drug Delivery Systems

The redox potential between the normal tissue and tumor tissue has been recently used in the delivery of anticancer drugs to the tumor tissue. The level of glutathione (GSH) plays an important role in regulation of cellular redox environment and is responsible for susceptibility and resistance to oxidative stress [133]. An increase in the glutathione level leads to an increase in the antioxidant capacity and oxidative stress resistance of cell, whereas a decrease in GSH level leads to an increase in susceptibility to oxidative stress. Consequently, the intracellular glutathione may act as a potential stimulus to stimulate the release of drug from the carrier system. GSH acts as a reducing agent which is present in cytosol, nucleus and mitochondria. The concentration of GSH in blood is less as compared to concentration of GSH in extracellular matrix, resulting in higher redox potential difference initiated by GSH, cysteine and other reducing agents. These reducing agents can help to induce breakage of the reducible bonds; which can destabilize the DDS leading to the release of therapeutic agents. The most cleavable bond is disulfide bond which has been introduced as a linker in the liposomes reduction [131]. Goldenbogen *et al.* (2011) synthesized the reduction sensitive doxorubicin entrapped liposomes and modified them with anti-HER2 antibody (tagged with biotin). Dithiothreitol, tris(2-carboxyethyl) phosphine, 1-cysteine and GSH caused the cleavage of disulfide bonds by eliminating the hydrophilic group of the conjugate, leading to the alteration of membrane organization and release of encapsulated drug [132].

Photosensitive Drug Delivery Systems

Light is an external stimulus which is used in the delivery of drugs. Light is used for the activation/inactivation of specific biochemical processes which is an effective technique for various biomedical applications. Various parameters like wavelength, intensity, pulse duration and cycle of activated light were used to modulate the light and used in biomedical research. Several radiations such as visible light, UV and near IR were clinically used in DDS. The near-infrared displayed deeper tissue penetration of drug in tumor cells [131]. The superficial tumor is mostly treated photodynamically which is a recognized tool for the management of superficial tumors. Photosensitizing agents, like chlorins, porphyrin derivatives, phthalocyanines and porphycenes are used for the diagnosis and treatment of cancer. These agents generate reactive oxygen radical species, which selectively destroy the targeted malignant tumor cells. The direct interaction (membrane fusion, photo-isomerism, photo fragmentation or photo polymerization) of liposomes with target cell occurs due to several photosensitive lipids (which provide the photo-triggered structural and conformational changes) [101, 131]. Zhu *et al.* (2012) prepared PEGylated liposomes containing benzo-porphyrin photosensitizers. Liposomes were modified with angiogenic endothelial cells specific peptide (Ala Pro Arg Pro Gly). The formulation showed higher growth inhibition of tumor cells [131].

Herbal Drug Approaches

Herbal medicines were used since ancient time when modern drugs were not discovered. The different synergistic combinations of plants were exploited for the treatment of innumerous diseases. Recently, new herbal drugs or combination of herbal drugs with conventional drugs are being investigated for their anticancer potential. Several studies were conducted throughout the world on herbal drugs development for the treatment of cancer [133]. The camptothecin analogues showed poor survival rate in patients of small cell lung cancer (SCLC). Therefore, the combination of camptothecin and capsaicin was investigated for the management of SCLC as a first line treatment. Capsaicin is herbal drug obtained from Capsicum frutescens and it enhanced the anticancer potential of conventional drug in animal models and cell lines. The results revealed the synergistic apoptosis response in classical and variant SCLC cells. The *in vivo* study was carried out in SCLC tumors xeno-transplanted on chicken chorioallantoic membrane models. The results demonstrated a synergistic response due to the enhancement of intracellular calcium and the calpain pathway [134]. Multidrug resistance (MDR) is the major drawback of conventional chemotherapy. The ABC (ATP binding cassette) pump was involved in resistance and drug efflux and decreased the intracellular drug concentration. The two herbal alkaloid drugs capsaicin and piperine were exploited for reversal of MDR in Caco-2 and CEM/ADR 5000 cell lines, which highly express P-glycoprotein (P-gp) and other ABC transporters. The biological source of capsaicin and piperine are *Capsicum frutescens* and *Piper nigrum*, respectively. The results of MTT study demonstrated that capsaicin and piperine increased the anticancer potential of doxorubicin. Rhodamine (Rho) 123 and calcein-AM were employed for confirming the activity of alkaloid on P-gp. The cytotoxicity of DOX was increased synergistically by this combination. These herbal drugs enhanced the accumulation of rhodamine and calcein (fluorescent substrates of P-gp) into the cell and avoided the efflux from the MDR cell lines. Capsaicin and piperine have chemo-sensitizing potential and combination of these drugs with chemotherapeutic agents improved the antitumor treatment efficiency [135]. The liposomal encapsulation of curcumin improved the anticancer efficiency, stability and reduced the toxicity. The preparation was characterized for various parameters like size, shape, surface charge, drug: lipid ratio and stability at 4 and 37 °C. The formulation with 0.05/10 drug-to-lipid molar ratio was stable and displayed 96% entrapment efficiency. Pancreatic adenocarcinoma (PA) is one of the most lethal type of cancers with low survival rate. Cancer metastasis was the major limiting factor affecting the treatment of cancer. Curcumin (Cur) is herbal agent which displayed potential antitumor property in PA but it has some drawbacks like low solubility, poor stability and limited bioavailability which limit its clinical use. Recently, nanotechnology based system have been exploited to overcome these drawbacks. The curcumin liposomes improved the cytotoxicity in the PA cancer cell lines AsPC-1 and BxPC-3 whereas, depicted less toxicity in normal cell line. Curcumin loaded liposomes also induced the apoptosis by generation of reactive oxygen species (ROS) and activation of caspase-3/7. The cell shrinkage, cytoplasmic blebbing and irregularity in shape morphological characters displayed the apoptosis potential. The liposomal formulation accumulated sufficient amount of curcumin into the tumor cell by enhanced permeability and retention effect and improved the treatment efficiency [136]. Polymeric nanoparticles (PNPs) were developed for the delivery of curcumin. The surface of PNPs was modified with chitosan and polyethylene glycol (PEG) which enhanced the circulation time and also improved the bioavailability of curcumin. Curcumin containing poly D,L-lactide-co-glycolide (PLGA) NPs coated with PEG and chitosan were prepared for the effective treatment of PA. The PNPs were having smooth surface, spherical in shape, nanometer in size and good loading efficiency. *In vitro* studies displayed better cytotoxicity, increased anti-migratory, anti-invasive and apoptosis-inducing capability of PNPs in metastatic PA [137]. A pentacyclic triterpenoid, Ursolic acid (UA), obtained from Hedyotis diffusa Willd, was studied for its antitumor potential in colon cancer, endometrial cancer and melanoma. Ursolic acid (UA) has good antitumor potential but its use is limited due to poor water-solubility and insufficient cellular uptake. The cationic nanomicelles were developed using Pluronic F127 and cationic C18-polyethylenimine (C18-PEI) polymer for the delivery of ursolic acid (UA) to colorectal cancer. The UA loaded micelles improved the inhibitory effects on cell viability as compared to free UA in colorectal cancer. The cationic nanomicelles arrested the cell cycle in G1 checkpoint and induced the apoptosis. The cell death due to apoptosis was analyzed using the annexin V antibody and propidium iodide staining. The results of western blot study demonstrated that regulation of Fas/FasL and activation of caspase-8 and caspase-3 was involved in apoptosis process [138]. *Tinospora cordifolia* is an ayurvedic herb utilized for the treatment of several diseases like gonorrhoea, diabetes, secondary syphilis, rheumatoid arthritis, anaemia, cancer, dermatological diseases, gout, asthma, jaundice, leprosy, *etc*. The component responsible for actual anticancer activity was investigated. The new clerodane diterpenoid, TC-2 triggered the ROS production and displayed the apoptosis inducing ability in colon cancer (HCT-116) cells. The clerodane furano diterpenoid also induced the autophagy in HCT116 cells. The outcomes revealed that autophagy and apoptosis were the major mechanisms responsible for anticancer activity. The activation of mitochondrial pathway, ROS production, release of cytochrome, nuclear fragmentation and caspase activation were the mechanisms involved in apoptosis [139]. The herbal drugs based novel drug delivery systems are depicted in Table **2**.

Table 2. Herbal drug based novel drug delivery systems.

System	Herbal Drug	Functionalizing Agent	Drug	Purpose	Refs.
Micelles	Resveratrol (RSV)	Folate	-	Breast cancer	[140]
GO-based nanocomposite	Berberine			pH and electrically controlled drug release	[141]
Chitosan nanoparticles	Ginsenoside compound K (CK)		-	Liver cancer	[142]
Polyamidoamine (PAMAM) dendrimer	Malloapelta B leaves of Mallotusapelta	Thermosensitive poly (N-isopropylacrylamide) (PNIPAM)	-	Liver cancer	[143]
Albumin nanocomposites	Berberine	Boronic acid	Etoposide	Lung cancer	[144]
Nanoparticles	Berberine (BER)	Lactoferrin (LF) and hyaluronic acid (HA)	Rapamycin (RAP)	Lung cancer	[145]
Liquid crystalline nanoparticles (LCNPs)	Aloe-emodin Aloe barbadensis Miller or Rheum palmatum	PEG	-	Breast cancer	[146]
Niosomes	Lawsone Persian Henna (Lawsoniainermis)			Breast cancer	[147]

(Table 2) cont.....

System	Herbal Drug	Functionalizing Agent	Drug	Purpose	Refs.
Single walled carbon nanotubes	Curcumin	Alginate (ALG) and chitosan (CHI)	-	Lung adenocarcinoma	[148]

CONCLUSION

Nanotechnology is an emerging field with high applicability in clinical areas like early diagnosis or disease treatment. Nanotechnology based systems such as liposomes, nanoparticles, hydogel and nanoemulsion were utilized for the delivery of various anticancer drugs. Further, the surface of carriers was modified with suitable ligand in order to enhance the delivery of drug in the neoplastic tissue. The conventional chemotherapy was invasive and non-specific in nature and also affects the normal cells. The targeted novel drug delivery systems modified with targeting agents improved the diagnosis and therapeutic potential of chemotherapeutic agents. Stimuli-triggered drug delivery systems offer a promising strategy to deliver and release drug in a site-specific manner. The unique features such as low pH of tumor microenvironment can serve as an endogenous stimulus to trigger the controlled release of drug in acidic medium. The various herbal agents have been exploited for their antitumor activity. The combination of natural agents with anticancer drugs showed synergistic response and reduced the dose as well as side effects of anticancer compounds. In clinical trials, nanotechnology based drug delivery systems meet many challenges such as lack of stability and efficiency, nonspecific immunogenicity, maintenance of controlled release of therapeutic molecules throughout the therapy. The chemical and surface modifications of nanocarriers are needed to overcome the problems of stability and nonspecific immunogenicity. Further modification with suitable targeting moiety is required for efficient and specific delivery. RNA therapeutics offer significant potential in clinical trials, while advanced targeting delivery approaches are needed for cancer therapy. The various types of modified nanocarriers such PEGylated, ligand conjugated, stimuli responsive (light, thermal, pH or magnetic) improved the precision, specificity and efficiency of anticancer agents due to selective delivery of drug to the target site. Further, suitable biochemical modifications may also improve the potency and reduce the toxic side effects, allowing the employment of new personalized drugs in clinical use.

CONSENT FOR PUBLICATION

Not applicable.

CONFLICT OF INTEREST

The authors confirm that this chapter contents have no conflict of interest.

ACKNOWLEDGEMENTS

Declared none.

REFERENCES

[1]   Hanahan D, Weinberg RA. Hallmarks of cancer: the next generation. Cell 2011; 144(5): 646-74.
        [http://dx.doi.org/10.1016/j.cell.2011.02.013] [PMID: 21376230]

[2]   Sharma VK, Jain A, Soni V. Nano-aggregates: emerging delivery tools for tumor therapy. Critical
        Reviews™ in Therapeutic Drug Carrier Systems 2013. 30(6): 535-63.
        [http://dx.doi.org/10.1615/CritRevTherDrugCarrierSyst.2013007706]

[3]   Chen F, Zhuang X, Lin L, *et al.* New horizons in tumor microenvironment biology: challenges and
        opportunities. BMC Med 2015; 13(1): 45.
        [http://dx.doi.org/10.1186/s12916-015-0278-7] [PMID: 25857315]

[4]   Gulbake A, Jain A, Jain A, Jain A, Jain SK. Insight to drug delivery aspects for colorectal cancer.
        World J Gastroenterol 2016; 22(2): 582-99.
        [http://dx.doi.org/10.3748/wjg.v22.i2.582] [PMID: 26811609]

[5]   Jain SK, Jain A. Ligand mediated drug targeted liposomes. Liposomal Delivery Systems: Advances
        and Challenges 2: Future Medicine Ltd Unitec House 2 Albert Place London N3 1QB UK. 2016; p.
        145.

[6]   Trédan O, Galmarini CM, Patel K, Tannock IF. Drug resistance and the solid tumor
        microenvironment. J Natl Cancer Inst 2007; 99(19): 1441-54.
        [http://dx.doi.org/10.1093/jnci/djm135] [PMID: 17895480]

[7]   Belli C, Trapani D, Viale G, *et al.* Targeting the microenvironment in solid tumors. Cancer Treat Rev
        2018; 65: 22-32.
        [http://dx.doi.org/10.1016/j.ctrv.2018.02.004] [PMID: 29502037]

[8]   Peer D, Karp JM, Hong S, Farokhzad OC, Margalit R, Langer R. Nanocarriers as an emerging
        platform for cancer therapy. Nat Nanotechnol 2007; 2(12): 751-60.
        [http://dx.doi.org/10.1038/nnano.2007.387] [PMID: 18654426]

[9]   Malam Y, Loizidou M, Seifalian AM. Liposomes and nanoparticles: nanosized vehicles for drug
        delivery in cancer. Trends Pharmacol Sci 2009; 30(11): 592-9.
        [http://dx.doi.org/10.1016/j.tips.2009.08.004] [PMID: 19837467]

[10]   Jain AJ, Jain SK. Liposomes in Cancer Therapy. In: Jimenez C, Ed. Nanocarrier Systems for Drug
        Delivery. New York: Nova Science Publishers 2016; pp. 1-42.

[11]   Cho K, Wang X, Nie S, Chen ZG, Shin DM. Therapeutic nanoparticles for drug delivery in cancer.
        Clin Cancer Res 2008; 14(5): 1310-6.
        [http://dx.doi.org/10.1158/1078-0432.CCR-07-1441] [PMID: 18316549]

[12]   Yezhelyev MV, Gao X, Xing Y, Al-Hajj A, Nie S, O'Regan RM. Emerging use of nanoparticles in
        diagnosis and treatment of breast cancer. Lancet Oncol 2006; 7(8): 657-67.
        [http://dx.doi.org/10.1016/S1470-2045(06)70793-8] [PMID: 16887483]

[13]   Jain A, Jain SK. Ligand-appended BBB-targeted nanocarriers (LABTNs). Critical Reviews™ in
        Therapeutic Drug Carrier Systems 2015; 32(2): 149-80.

[14]   Verma A, Sharma G, Jain A, *et al.* Systematic optimization of cationic surface engineered
        mucoadhesive vesicles employing Design of Experiment (DoE): A preclinical investigation. Int J Biol

Macromol 2019; 133: 1142-55.
[http://dx.doi.org/10.1016/j.ijbiomac.2019.04.118] [PMID: 31004631]

[15]   Ferrari M. Cancer nanotechnology: opportunities and challenges. Nat Rev Cancer 2005; 5(3): 161-71.
[http://dx.doi.org/10.1038/nrc1566] [PMID: 15738981]

[16]   Brigger I, Dubernet C, Couvreur P. Nanoparticles in cancer therapy and diagnosis. Adv Drug Deliv
Rev 2012; 64: 24-36.
[http://dx.doi.org/10.1016/j.addr.2012.09.006] [PMID: 12204596]

[17]   Jain A, Kumari R, Tiwari A, *et al.* Nanocarrier based advances in drug delivery to tumor: an overview.
Curr Drug Targets 2018; 19(13): 1498-518.
[http://dx.doi.org/10.2174/1389450119666180131105822] [PMID: 29384060]

[18]   Sutradhar KB, Amin ML. Nanotechnology in cancer drug delivery and selective targeting. 2014: 1-12.
[http://dx.doi.org/10.1155/2014/939378]

[19]   Lale SV, Koul V. Stimuli-Responsive Polymeric Nanoparticles for Cancer. Therapy. Polymer Gels:
Springer 2018; pp. 27-54.

[20]   Jain A, Jain SK. Stimuli-responsive Smart Liposomes in Cancer Targeting. Curr Drug Targets 2018;
19(3): 259-70.
[http://dx.doi.org/10.2174/1389450117666160208144143] [PMID: 26853324]

[21]   Figueiredo P, Bauleth-Ramos T, Hirvonen J, Sarmento B, Santos HA. The Emerging Role of
Multifunctional Theranostic Materials in Cancer Nanomedicine Handbook of Nanomaterials for
Cancer Theranostics. Elsevier 2018; pp. 1-31.

[22]   Wicki A, Witzigmann D, Balasubramanian V, Huwyler J. Nanomedicine in cancer therapy:
challenges, opportunities, and clinical applications. J Control Release 2015; 200: 138-57.
[http://dx.doi.org/10.1016/j.jconrel.2014.12.030] [PMID: 25545217]

[23]   Jokerst JV, Gambhir SS. Molecular imaging with theranostic nanoparticles. Acc Chem Res 2011;
44(10): 1050-60.
[http://dx.doi.org/10.1021/ar200106e] [PMID: 21919457]

[24]   Jain A, Jain SK. Colon Targeted Liposomal Systems (CTLS): Theranostic Potential. Curr Mol Med
2015; 15(7): 621-33. [eng.].
[http://dx.doi.org/10.2174/1566524015666150831131320] [PMID: 26321756]

[25]   Al-Jamal WT, Kostarelos K. Liposomes: from a clinically established drug delivery system to a
nanoparticle platform for theranostic nanomedicine. Acc Chem Res 2011; 44(10): 1094-104.
[http://dx.doi.org/10.1021/ar200105p] [PMID: 21812415]

[26]   Sanjay Kumar J, Ankita T, Ankit J, Amit V, Shivani S, Pritish Kumar P, *et al.* Application Potential of
Polymeric Nanoconstructs for Colon-Specific Drug Delivery Multifunctional Nanocarriers for
Contemporary Healthcare Applications. Hershey, PA, USA: IGI Global 2018; pp. 22-49.

[27]   Prajapati SK, Jain A, Shrivastava C, Jain AK. Hyaluronic acid conjugated multi-walled carbon
nanotubes for colon cancer targeting. Int J Biol Macromol 2019; 123: 691-703.
[http://dx.doi.org/10.1016/j.ijbiomac.2018.11.116]

[28]   Hou L, Shan X, Hao L, Feng Q, Zhang Z. Copper sulfide nanoparticle-based localized drug delivery
system as an effective cancer synergistic treatment and theranostic platform. Acta Biomater 2017; 54:
307-20.
[http://dx.doi.org/10.1016/j.actbio.2017.03.005] [PMID: 28274767]

[29]   Patitsa M, Karathanou K, Kanaki Z, *et al.* Magnetic nanoparticles coated with polyarabic acid
demonstrate enhanced drug delivery and imaging properties for cancer theranostic applications. Sci
Rep 2017; 7(1): 775.
[http://dx.doi.org/10.1038/s41598-017-00836-y] [PMID: 28396592]

[30]   Ko N, Nafiujjaman M, Lee J, Lim H-N, Lee Y-k, Kwon I. Graphene quantum dot-based theranostic

agents for active targeting of breast cancer. RSC Advances 2017; 7(19): 11420-7.
[http://dx.doi.org/10.1039/C6RA25949A]

[31]   Lin C-J, Kuan C-H, Wang L-W, *et al*. Integrated self-assembling drug delivery system possessing dual
responsive and active targeting for orthotopic ovarian cancer theranostics. Biomaterials 2016; 90: 12-
26.
[http://dx.doi.org/10.1016/j.biomaterials.2016.03.005] [PMID: 26974704]

[32]   Muthu MS, Kutty RV, Luo Z, Xie J, Feng S-S. Theranostic vitamin E TPGS micelles of transferrin
conjugation for targeted co-delivery of docetaxel and ultra bright gold nanoclusters. Biomaterials
2015; 39: 234-48.
[http://dx.doi.org/10.1016/j.biomaterials.2014.11.008] [PMID: 25468374]

[33]   Wang L, Zhang H, Qin A, Jin Q, Tang BZ, Ji J. Theranostic hyaluronic acid prodrug micelles with
aggregation-induced emission characteristics for targeted drug delivery. Sci China Chem 2016; 59(12):
1609-15.
[http://dx.doi.org/10.1007/s11426-016-0246-9]

[34]   Bwatanglang IB, Mohammad F, Yusof NA, *et al*. Folic acid targeted Mn:ZnS quantum dots for
theranostic applications of cancer cell imaging and therapy. Int J Nanomedicine 2016; 11: 413-28.
[PMID: 26858524]

[35]   Flores O, Santra S, Kaittanis C, *et al*. PSMA-targeted theranostic nanocarrier for prostate cancer.
Theranostics 2017; 7(9): 2477-94.
[http://dx.doi.org/10.7150/thno.18879] [PMID: 28744329]

[36]   Patel NR, Piroyan A, Ganta S, *et al*. *In vitro* and *in vivo* evaluation of a novel folate-targeted
theranostic nanoemulsion of docetaxel for imaging and improved anticancer activity against ovarian
cancers. Cancer Biol Ther 2018; 19(7): 554-64.
[http://dx.doi.org/10.1080/15384047.2017.1395118] [PMID: 29737910]

[37]   Gao N, Bozeman EN, Qian W, *et al*. Tumor penetrating theranostic nanoparticles for enhancement of
targeted and image-guided drug delivery into peritoneal tumors following intraperitoneal delivery.
Theranostics 2017; 7(6): 1689-704.
[http://dx.doi.org/10.7150/thno.18125] [PMID: 28529645]

[38]   Jain A, Jain SK. Application potential of engineered liposomes in tumor targeting.Multifunctional
Systems for Combined Delivery, Biosensing and Diagnostics. Elsevier - Health Sciences Division
2017; pp. 171-92.
[http://dx.doi.org/10.1016/B978-0-323-52725-5.00009-5]

[39]   Jain A, Jain SK. Multipronged, strategic delivery of paclitaxel-topotecan using engineered liposomes
to ovarian cancer. Drug Dev Ind Pharm 2016; 42(1): 136-49.
[http://dx.doi.org/10.3109/03639045.2015.1036066] [PMID: 26006330]

[40]   Jain A, Gulbake A, Jain A, Shilpi S, Hurkat P, Jain SK. Dual drug delivery using "smart" liposomes
for triggered release of anticancer agents. J Nanopart Res 2013; 15(7): 1772.
[http://dx.doi.org/10.1007/s11051-013-1772-5]

[41]   Jain A, Hurkat P, Jain SK. Development of liposomes using formulation by design: Basics to recent
advances. Chem Phys Lipids 2019; •••S0009-3084(18)30081-1
[http://dx.doi.org/10.1016/j.chemphyslip.2019.03.017] [PMID: 30951713]

[42]   Peres-Filho MJ, Dos Santos AP, Nascimento TL, *et al*. Antiproliferative Activity and VEGF
Expression Reduction in MCF7 and PC-3 Cancer Cells by Paclitaxel and Imatinib Co-encapsulation in
Folate-Targeted Liposomes. AAPS PharmSciTech 2018; 19(1): 201-12.
[http://dx.doi.org/10.1208/s12249-017-0830-1] [PMID: 28681330]

[43]   Zhang L-X, Li K-F, Wang H, *et al*. Preparation and *in vitro* evaluation of a MRI contrast agent based
on aptamer-modified gadolinium-loaded liposomes for tumor targeting. AAPS PharmSciTech 2017;
18(5): 1564-71.
[http://dx.doi.org/10.1208/s12249-016-0600-5] [PMID: 27604884]

[44]   Kang JH, Battogtokh G, Ko YT. Folate-targeted liposome encapsulating chitosan/oligonucleotide polyplexes for tumor targeting. AAPS PharmSciTech 2014; 15(5): 1087-92.
        [http://dx.doi.org/10.1208/s12249-014-0136-5] [PMID: 24848761]

[45]   Hu T, Cao H, Yang C, *et al.* LHD-modified mechanism-based liposome coencapsulation of mitoxantrone and prednisolone using novel lipid bilayer fusion for tissue-specific colocalization and synergistic antitumor effects. ACS Appl Mater Interfaces 2016; 8(10): 6586-601.
        [http://dx.doi.org/10.1021/acsami.5b10598] [PMID: 26907854]

[46]   Pirollo KF, Nemunaitis J, Leung PK, Nunan R, Adams J, Chang EH. Safety and Efficacy in Advanced Solid Tumors of a Targeted Nanocomplex Carrying the p53 Gene Used in Combination with Docetaxel: A Phase 1b Study. Mol Ther 2016; 24(9): 1697-706. [eng.].
        [http://dx.doi.org/10.1038/mt.2016.135] [PMID: 27357628]

[47]   Siefker-Radtke A, Zhang XQ, Guo CC, *et al.* A phase 1 study of a tumor-targeted systemic nanodelivery system, SGT-94, in genitourinary cancers. Mol Ther 2016; 24(8): 1484-91.
        [http://dx.doi.org/10.1038/mt.2016.118] [PMID: 27480598]

[48]   Dangi R, Hurkat P, Jain A, *et al.* Targeting liver cancer *via* ASGP receptor using 5-FU-loaded surface-modified PLGA nanoparticles. J Microencapsul 2014; 31(5): 479-87.
        [http://dx.doi.org/10.3109/02652048.2013.879929] [PMID: 24697169]

[49]   Graziani SR, Vital CG, Morikawa AT, *et al.* Phase II study of paclitaxel associated with lipid core nanoparticles (LDE) as third-line treatment of patients with epithelial ovarian carcinoma. Med Oncol 2017; 34(9): 151.
        [http://dx.doi.org/10.1007/s12032-017-1009-z] [PMID: 28756613]

[50]   Pham E, Birrer MJ, Eliasof S, *et al.* Translational impact of nanoparticle-drug conjugate CRLX101 with or without bevacizumab in advanced ovarian cancer. Clin Cancer Res 2015; 21(4): 808-18.
        [http://dx.doi.org/clincanres. 2810.014]

[51]   López-Viota M, El-Hammadi MM, Cabeza L, *et al.* Development and Characterization of Magnetite/Poly(butylcyanoacrylate) Nanoparticles for Magnetic Targeted Delivery of Cancer Drugs. AAPS PharmSciTech 2017; 18(8): 3042-52.
        [http://dx.doi.org/10.1208/s12249-017-0792-3] [PMID: 28508129]

[52]   Sun Y, Zhang J, Han J, *et al.* Galactose-Containing Polymer-DOX Conjugates for Targeting Drug Delivery. AAPS PharmSciTech 2017; 18(3): 749-58.
        [http://dx.doi.org/10.1208/s12249-016-0557-4] [PMID: 27287244]

[53]   Zhao H, Yuan X, Yu J, *et al.* Magnesium-Stabilized Multifunctional DNA Nanoparticles for Tumor-Targeted and pH-Responsive Drug Delivery. ACS Appl Mater Interfaces 2018; 10(18): 15418-27.
        [http://dx.doi.org/10.1021/acsami.8b01932] [PMID: 29676144]

[54]   Gianella A, Jarzyna PA, Mani V, *et al.* Multifunctional nanoemulsion platform for imaging guided therapy evaluated in experimental cancer. ACS Nano 2011; 5(6): 4422-33.
        [http://dx.doi.org/10.1021/nn103336a] [PMID: 21557611]

[55]   Yadav S, Gupta S. Development and *in vitro* characterization of docetaxel-loaded ligand appended solid fat nanoemulsions for potential use in breast cancer therapy. Artif Cells Nanomed Biotechnol 2015; 43(2): 93-102. [eng.].
        [http://dx.doi.org/10.3109/21691401.2013.845569] [PMID: 24195582]

[56]   Kim J-E, Park Y-J. Improved antitumor efficacy of hyaluronic acid-complexed paclitaxel nanoemulsions in treating non-small cell lung cancer. Biomol Ther (Seoul) 2017; 25(4): 411-6.
        [http://dx.doi.org/10.4062/biomolther.2016.261] [PMID: 28208014]

[57]   Jain A, Jain SK. Environmentally Responsive Chitosan-based Nanocarriers (CBNs). Handbook of Polymers for Pharmaceutical Technologies, Biodegradable Polymers. 2015; 3: p. 105.

[58]   Hansen TD, Koepsel JT, Le NN, *et al.* Biomaterial arrays with defined adhesion ligand densities and matrix stiffness identify distinct phenotypes for tumorigenic and nontumorigenic human mesenchymal

cell types. Biomater Sci 2014; 2(5): 745-56.
[http://dx.doi.org/10.1039/C3BM60278H] [PMID: 25386339]

[59]   Li X, Xiulan S. Multifunctional smart hydrogels: potential in tissue engineering and cancer therapy. J
        Mater Chem B Mater Biol Med 2018; 6: 4714-30.
        [http://dx.doi.org/10.1039/C8TB01078A]

[60]   Zhu X, Zhang H, Huang H, Zhang Y, Hou L, Zhang Z. Functionalized graphene oxide-based
        thermosensitive hydrogel for magnetic hyperthermia therapy on tumors. Nanotechnology 2015;
        26(36): 365103.
        [http://dx.doi.org/10.1088/0957-4484/26/36/365103] [PMID: 26291977]

[61]   Karavasili C, Panteris E, Vizirianakis IS, Koutsopoulos S, Fatouros DG. Chemotherapeutic Delivery
        from a Self-Assembling Peptide Nanofiber Hydrogel for the Management of Glioblastoma. Pharm Res
        2018; 35(8): 166.
        [http://dx.doi.org/10.1007/s11095-018-2442-1] [PMID: 29943122]

[62]   Makhmalzadeh BS, Molavi O, Vakili MR, *et al.* Functionalized Caprolactone-Polyethylene Glycol
        Based Thermo-Responsive Hydrogels of Silibinin for the Treatment of Malignant Melanoma. J Pharm
        Pharm Sci 2018; 21(1): 143-59.
        [http://dx.doi.org/10.18433/jpps29726] [PMID: 29789104]

[63]   Trimble CL, Morrow MP, Kraynyak KA, *et al.* Safety, efficacy, and immunogenicity of VGX-3100, a
        therapeutic synthetic DNA vaccine targeting human papillomavirus 16 and 18 E6 and E7 proteins for
        cervical intraepithelial neoplasia 2/3: a randomised, double-blind, placebo-controlled phase 2b trial.
        Lancet 2015; 386(10008): 2078-88.
        [http://dx.doi.org/10.1016/S0140-6736(15)00239-1] [PMID: 26386540]

[64]   Russell SJ, Peng K-W. Oncolytic virotherapy: a contest between apples and oranges. Mol Ther 2017;
        25(5): 1107-16.
        [http://dx.doi.org/10.1016/j.ymthe.2017.03.026] [PMID: 28392162]

[65]   Husain SR, Han J, Au P, Shannon K, Puri RK. Gene therapy for cancer: regulatory considerations for
        approval. Cancer Gene Ther 2015; 22(12): 554-63.
        [http://dx.doi.org/10.1038/cgt.2015.58] [PMID: 26584531]

[66]   Morita Y, Leslie M, Kameyama H, Volk DE, Tanaka T. Aptamer Therapeutics in Cancer: Current and
        Future. Cancers (Basel) 2018; 10(3): 80.
        [http://dx.doi.org/10.3390/cancers10030080] [PMID: 29562664]

[67]   Yuan B, Jiang X, Chen Y, *et al.* Metastatic cancer cell and tissue-specific fluorescence imaging using
        a new DNA aptamer developed by Cell-SELEX. Talanta 2017; 170: 56-62.
        [http://dx.doi.org/10.1016/j.talanta.2017.03.094] [PMID: 28501211]

[68]   Duan M, Long Y, Yang C, *et al.* Selection and characterization of DNA aptamer for metastatic
        prostate cancer recognition and tissue imaging. Oncotarget 2016; 7(24): 36436-46.
        [http://dx.doi.org/10.18632/oncotarget.9262] [PMID: 27183906]

[69]   Chen H, Yuan C-H, Yang Y-F, Yin C-Q, Guan Q, Wang F-B, *et al.* Subtractive cell-SELEX selection
        of DNA aptamers binding specifically and selectively to hepatocellular carcinoma cells with high
        metastatic potential. BioMed research international 2016(1): 1-9.
        [http://dx.doi.org/10.1155/2016/5735869]

[70]   Kryza D, Debordeaux F, Azéma L, *et al. Ex vivo* and *in vivo* imaging and biodistribution of aptamers
        targeting the human matrix metalloprotease-9 in melanomas. PLoS One 2016; 11(2): e0149387.
        [http://dx.doi.org/10.1371/journal.pone.0149387] [PMID: 26901393]

[71]   Li K, Xiu CL, Gao LM, *et al.* Screening of specific nucleic acid aptamers binding tumor markers in
        the serum of the lung cancer patients and identification of their activities. Tumour Biol 2017; 39(7):
        1010428317717123.
        [http://dx.doi.org/10.1177/1010428317717123] [PMID: 28718373]

[72]   Tsai S-C, Hung L-Y, Lee G-B. An integrated microfluidic system for the isolation and detection of ovarian circulating tumor cells using cell selection and enrichment methods. Biomicrofluidics 2017; 11(3): 034122.
[http://dx.doi.org/10.1063/1.4991476] [PMID: 28713478]

[73]   Rosenberg JE, Bambury RM, Van Allen EM, *et al.* A phase II trial of AS1411 (a novel nucleolin-targeted DNA aptamer) in metastatic renal cell carcinoma. Invest New Drugs 2014; 32(1): 178-87.
[http://dx.doi.org/10.1007/s10637-013-0045-6] [PMID: 24242861]

[74]   Vater A, Klussmann S. Toward third-generation aptamers: Spiegelmers and their therapeutic prospects. Curr Opin Drug Discov Devel 2003; 6(2): 253-61.
[PMID: 12669461]

[75]   Vater A, Sahlmann J, Kröger N, *et al.* Hematopoietic stem and progenitor cell mobilization in mice and humans by a first-in-class mirror-image oligonucleotide inhibitor of CXCL12. Clin Pharmacol Ther 2013; 94(1): 150-7.
[http://dx.doi.org/10.1038/clpt.2013.58] [PMID: 23588307]

[76]   Rettig WJ, Old LJ. Immunogenetics of human cell surface differentiation. Annu Rev Immunol 1989; 7(1): 481-511.
[http://dx.doi.org/10.1146/annurev.iy.07.040189.002405] [PMID: 2653374]

[77]   Maloney DG, Grillo-López AJ, White CA, *et al.* IDEC-C2B8 (Rituximab) anti-CD20 monoclonal antibody therapy in patients with relapsed low-grade non-Hodgkin's lymphoma. Blood 1997; 90(6): 2188-95.
[PMID: 9310469]

[78]   Beers SA, Chan CH, French RR, Cragg MS, Glennie MJ, Eds. CD20 as a target for therapeutic type I and II monoclonal antibodies Semin Hematol. Elsevier 2010.

[79]   Witzig TE, Flinn IW, Gordon LI, *et al.* Treatment with ibritumomab tiuxetan radioimmunotherapy in patients with rituximab-refractory follicular non-Hodgkin's lymphoma. J Clin Oncol 2002; 20(15): 3262-9.
[http://dx.doi.org/10.1200/JCO.2002.11.017] [PMID: 12149300]

[80]   Skarbnik AP, Smith MR. Radioimmunotherapy in mantle cell lymphoma. Best Pract Res Clin Haematol 2012; 25(2): 201-10.
[http://dx.doi.org/10.1016/j.beha.2012.04.004] [PMID: 22687456]

[81]   Tobinai K, Klein C, Oya N, Fingerle-Rowson G. A review of obinutuzumab (GA101), a novel type II anti-CD20 monoclonal antibody, for the treatment of patients with B-cell malignancies. Adv Ther 2017; 34(2): 324-56.
[http://dx.doi.org/10.1007/s12325-016-0451-1] [PMID: 28004361]

[82]   Goldenberg DM, Morschhauser F, Wegener WA. Veltuzumab (humanized anti-CD20 monoclonal antibody): characterization, current clinical results, and future prospects. Leuk Lymphoma 2010; 51(5): 747-55.
[http://dx.doi.org/10.3109/10428191003672123] [PMID: 20214444]

[83]   Robak T, Robak E. New anti-CD20 monoclonal antibodies for the treatment of B-cell lymphoid malignancies. BioDrugs 2011; 25(1): 13-25.
[http://dx.doi.org/10.2165/11539590-000000000-00000] [PMID: 21090841]

[84]   Hu Y, Turner MJ, Shields J, *et al.* Investigation of the mechanism of action of alemtuzumab in a human CD52 transgenic mouse model. Immunology 2009; 128(2): 260-70.
[http://dx.doi.org/10.1111/j.1365-2567.2009.03115.x] [PMID: 19740383]

[85]   Christian BA, Poi M, Jones JA, *et al.* The combination of milatuzumab, a humanized anti-CD74 antibody, and veltuzumab, a humanized anti-CD20 antibody, demonstrates activity in patients with relapsed and refractory B-cell non-Hodgkin lymphoma. Br J Haematol 2015; 169(5): 701-10.
[http://dx.doi.org/10.1111/bjh.13354] [PMID: 25847298]

[86]   Lambert JM. Drug-conjugated monoclonal antibodies for the treatment of cancer. Curr Opin Pharmacol 2005; 5(5): 543-9.
[http://dx.doi.org/10.1016/j.coph.2005.04.017] [PMID: 16087399]

[87]   Alley SC, Okeley NM, Senter PD. Antibody-drug conjugates: targeted drug delivery for cancer. Curr Opin Chem Biol 2010; 14(4): 529-37.
[http://dx.doi.org/10.1016/j.cbpa.2010.06.170] [PMID: 20643572]

[88]   Peddi PF, Hurvitz SA. Trastuzumab emtansine: the first targeted chemotherapy for treatment of breast cancer. Future Oncol 2013; 9(3): 319-26.
[http://dx.doi.org/10.2217/fon.13.7] [PMID: 23469968]

[89]   Jager E, van der Velden VH, te Marvelde JG, Walter RB, Agur Z, Vainstein V. Targeted drug delivery by gemtuzumab ozogamicin: mechanism-based mathematical model for treatment strategy improvement and therapy individualization. PLoS One 2011; 6(9): e24265.
[http://dx.doi.org/10.1371/journal.pone.0024265] [PMID: 21915304]

[90]   Bhatt S, Ashlock BM, Natkunam Y, Sujoy V, Chapman JR, Ramos JC, *et al.* CD30 targeting with brentuximab vedotin: a novel therapeutic approach to primary effusion lymphoma. Blood 2013. blood-2013-01-481713.
[http://dx.doi.org/10.1182/blood-2013-01-481713]

[91]   Kantarjian H, Thomas D, Jorgensen J, *et al.* Results of inotuzumab ozogamicin, a CD22 monoclonal antibody, in refractory and relapsed acute lymphocytic leukemia. Cancer 2013; 119(15): 2728-36.
[http://dx.doi.org/10.1002/cncr.28136] [PMID: 23633004]

[92]   Whiteman KR, Johnson HA, Mayo MF, Audette CA, Carrigan CN, LaBelle A, Eds. Lorvotuzumab mertansine, a CD56-targeting antibody-drug conjugate with potent antitumor activity against small cell lung cancer in human xenograft models MAbs. Taylor & Francis 2014.
[http://dx.doi.org/10.4161/mabs.27756]

[93]   Yang K, Feng L, Liu Z. Stimuli responsive drug delivery systems based on nano-graphene for cancer therapy. Adv Drug Deliv Rev 2016; 105(Pt B): 228-41.
[http://dx.doi.org/10.1016/j.addr.2016.05.015] [PMID: 27233212]

[94]   Xiao W, Zeng X, Lin H, Han K, Jia H-Z, Zhang X-Z. Dual stimuli-responsive multi-drug delivery system for the individually controlled release of anti-cancer drugs. Chem Commun (Camb) 2015; 51(8): 1475-8.
[http://dx.doi.org/10.1039/C4CC08831J] [PMID: 25494173]

[95]   Luo D, Carter KA, Razi A, *et al.* Doxorubicin encapsulated in stealth liposomes conferred with light-triggered drug release. Biomaterials 2016; 75: 193-202.
[http://dx.doi.org/10.1016/j.biomaterials.2015.10.027] [PMID: 26513413]

[96]   Zheng F-F, Zhang P-H, Xi Y, Chen J-J, Li L-L, Zhu J-J. Aptamer/graphene quantum dots nanocomposite capped fluorescent mesoporous silica nanoparticles for intracellular drug delivery and real-time monitoring of drug release. Anal Chem 2015; 87(23): 11739-45.
[http://dx.doi.org/10.1021/acs.analchem.5b03131] [PMID: 26524192]

[97]   Paris JL, Cabañas MV, Manzano M, Vallet-Regí M. Polymer-grafted mesoporous silica nanoparticles as ultrasound-responsive drug carriers. ACS Nano 2015; 9(11): 11023-33.
[http://dx.doi.org/10.1021/acsnano.5b04378] [PMID: 26456489]

[98]   Jin S, Wan J, Meng L, *et al.* Biodegradation and toxicity of protease/redox/pH stimuli-responsive PEGlated PMAA nanohydrogels for targeting drug delivery. ACS Appl Mater Interfaces 2015; 7(35): 19843-52.
[http://dx.doi.org/10.1021/acsami.5b05984] [PMID: 26288386]

[99]   Hwang AA, Lee BY, Clemens DL, Dillon BJ, Zink JI, Horwitz MA. pH-Responsive Isoniazid-Loaded Nanoparticles Markedly Improve Tuberculosis Treatment in Mice. Small 2015; 11(38): 5066-78.
[http://dx.doi.org/10.1002/smll.201500937] [PMID: 26193431]

[100]   Du J, Lane LA, Nie S. Stimuli-responsive nanoparticles for targeting the tumor microenvironment. J Control Release 2015; 219: 205-14.
[http://dx.doi.org/10.1016/j.jconrel.2015.08.050] [PMID: 26341694]

[101]   Torchilin VP. Targeted pharmaceutical nanocarriers for cancer therapy and imaging. AAPS J 2007; 9(2): E128-47.
[http://dx.doi.org/10.1208/aapsj0902015] [PMID: 17614355]

[102]   Jain A, Tiwari A, Verma A, Jain SK. Ultrasound-based triggered drug delivery to tumors. Drug Deliv Transl Res 2017; 1-15.
[PMID: 29204925]

[103]   Jain A, Jain SK. *In vitro* release kinetics model fitting of liposomes: An insight. Chem Phys Lipids 2016; 201: 28-40.
[http://dx.doi.org/10.1016/j.chemphyslip.2016.10.005] [PMID: 27983957]

[104]   Zhang W, Gao C. Recent advances in cell imaging and cytotoxicity of intracellular stimuli-responsive nanomaterials. Sci Bull (Beijing) 2015; 60(23): 1973-9.
[http://dx.doi.org/10.1007/s11434-015-0952-3]

[105]   Zhao Y. Sensing system for mimicking cancer cell–drug interaction. Sci Bull (Beijing) 2015; 60(13): 1218-9.
[http://dx.doi.org/10.1007/s11434-015-0835-7]

[106]   Das D, Ghosh P, Ghosh A, *et al.* Stimulus-responsive, biodegradable, biocompatible, covalently cross-linked hydrogel based on dextrin and poly (N-isopropylacrylamide) for *in vitro/in vivo* controlled drug release. ACS Appl Mater Interfaces 2015; 7(26): 14338-51.
[http://dx.doi.org/10.1021/acsami.5b02975] [PMID: 26069986]

[107]   Langer R. Where a pill won't reach. Sci Am 2003; 288(4): 50-7.
[http://dx.doi.org/10.1038/scientificamerican0403-50] [PMID: 12661315]

[108]   Hu H, Yu J, Li Y, Zhao J, Dong H. Engineering of a novel pluronic F127/graphene nanohybrid for pH responsive drug delivery. J Biomed Mater Res A 2012; 100(1): 141-8.
[http://dx.doi.org/10.1002/jbm.a.33252] [PMID: 21997951]

[109]   Kale AA, Torchilin VP. Environment-responsive multifunctional liposomes Liposomes. Springer 2010; pp. 213-42.

[110]   Danhier F, Feron O, Préat V. To exploit the tumor microenvironment: Passive and active tumor targeting of nanocarriers for anti-cancer drug delivery. J Control Release 2010; 148(2): 135-46. [eng.].
[http://dx.doi.org/10.1016/j.jconrel.2010.08.027] [PMID: 20797419]

[111]   Arias JL, Clares B, Morales ME, Gallardo V, Ruiz MA. Lipid-based drug delivery systems for cancer treatment. Curr Drug Targets 2011; 12(8): 1151-65. [eng.].
[http://dx.doi.org/10.2174/138945011795906570] [PMID: 21443475]

[112]   Deshpande PP, Biswas S, Torchilin VP. Current trends in the use of liposomes for tumor targeting. Nanomedicine (Lond) 2013; 8(9): 1509-28.
[http://dx.doi.org/10.2217/nnm.13.118] [PMID: 23914966]

[113]   Goenka S, Sant V, Sant S. Graphene-based nanomaterials for drug delivery and tissue engineering. J Control Release 2014; 173: 75-88.
[http://dx.doi.org/10.1016/j.jconrel.2013.10.017] [PMID: 24161530]

[114]   Yu J, Chu X, Hou Y. Stimuli-responsive cancer therapy based on nanoparticles. Chem Commun (Camb) 2014; 50(79): 11614-30.
[http://dx.doi.org/10.1039/C4CC03984J] [PMID: 25058003]

[115]   He X, Li J, An S, Jiang C. pH-sensitive drug-delivery systems for tumor targeting. Ther Deliv 2013; 4(12): 1499-510.
[http://dx.doi.org/10.4155/tde.13.120] [PMID: 24304248]

[116]   Saraf S, Jain A, Hurkat P, Jain SK. Topotecan Liposomes: A Visit from a Molecular to a Therapeutic Platform. Crit Rev Ther Drug Carrier Syst 2016; 33(5): 401-32.
[http://dx.doi.org/10.1615/CritRevTherDrugCarrierSyst.2016015926] [PMID: 27910741]

[117]   Crayton SH, Tsourkas A. pH-titratable superparamagnetic iron oxide for improved nanoparticle accumulation in acidic tumor microenvironments. ACS Nano 2011; 5(12): 9592-601.
[http://dx.doi.org/10.1021/nn202863x] [PMID: 22035454]

[118]   Zhou T, Zhou X, Xing D. Controlled release of doxorubicin from graphene oxide based charge-reversal nanocarrier. Biomaterials 2014; 35(13): 4185-94.
[http://dx.doi.org/10.1016/j.biomaterials.2014.01.044] [PMID: 24513318]

[119]   Feng L, Li K, Shi X, Gao M, Liu J, Liu Z. Smart pH-responsive nanocarriers based on nano-graphene oxide for combined chemo- and photothermal therapy overcoming drug resistance. Adv Healthc Mater 2014; 3(8): 1261-71.
[http://dx.doi.org/10.1002/adhm.201300549] [PMID: 24652715]

[120]   Liu J, Huang Y, Kumar A, *et al.* pH-sensitive nano-systems for drug delivery in cancer therapy. Biotechnol Adv 2014; 32(4): 693-710.
[http://dx.doi.org/10.1016/j.biotechadv.2013.11.009] [PMID: 24309541]

[121]   Ke CJ, Su TY, Chen HL, *et al.* Smart multifunctional hollow microspheres for the quick release of drugs in intracellular lysosomal compartments. Angew Chem Int Ed Engl 2011; 50(35): 8086-9.
[http://dx.doi.org/10.1002/anie.201102852] [PMID: 21751316]

[122]   Ramos J, Imaz A, Forcada J. Temperature-sensitive nanogels: poly (N-vinylcaprolactam) versus poly (N-isopropylacrylamide). Polym Chem 2012; 3(4): 852-6.
[http://dx.doi.org/10.1039/C2PY00485B]

[123]   Jadhav SA, Miletto I, Brunella V, Berlier G, Scalarone D. Controlled post□synthesis grafting of thermoresponsive poly (N□isopropylacrylamide) on mesoporous silica nanoparticles. Polym Adv Technol 2015; 26(9): 1070-5.
[http://dx.doi.org/10.1002/pat.3534]

[124]   Heo MS, Seo EJ, John JV, Jang IH, Kim JH, Kim I. Synthesis of hyperbranched polyglycidol--poly(N-isopropylacrylamide) using nitroxide-mediated polymerization for thermosensitive drug delivery system. J Control Release 2015; 213(213)e80
[http://dx.doi.org/10.1016/j.jconrel.2015.05.133] [PMID: 27005234]

[125]   Idziak I, Avoce D, Lessard D, Gravel D, Zhu X. Thermosensitivity of aqueous solutions of poly (N, N-diethylacrylamide). Macromolecules 1999; 32(4): 1260-3.
[http://dx.doi.org/10.1021/ma981171f]

[126]   Aoki T, Kawashima M, Katono H, Sanui K, Ogata N, Okano T, *et al.* Temperature-responsive interpenetrating polymer networks constructed with poly (acrylic acid) and poly (N, N-dimethylacrylamide). Macromolecules 1994; 27(4): 947-52.
[http://dx.doi.org/10.1021/ma00082a010]

[127]   Staruch RM, Hynynen K, Chopra R. Hyperthermia-mediated doxorubicin release from thermosensitive liposomes using MR-HIFU: therapeutic effect in rabbit Vx2 tumours. Int J Hyperthermia 2015; 31(2): 118-33.
[http://dx.doi.org/10.3109/02656736.2014.992483] [PMID: 25582131]

[128]   May JP, Li S-D. Hyperthermia-induced drug targeting. Expert Opin Drug Deliv 2013; 10(4): 511-27.
[http://dx.doi.org/10.1517/17425247.2013.758631] [PMID: 23289519]

[129]   Grüll H, Langereis S. Hyperthermia-triggered drug delivery from temperature-sensitive liposomes using MRI-guided high intensity focused ultrasound. J Control Release 2012; 161(2): 317-27. [eng.].
[http://dx.doi.org/10.1016/j.jconrel.2012.04.041] [PMID: 22565055]

[130]   Jhaveri A. Magnetic Field-Responsive Nanocarriers Smart Pharmaceutical Nanocarriers. World Scientific 2016; pp. 267-308.

[http://dx.doi.org/10.1142/9781783267231_0009]

[131]   Zhu L, Torchilin VP. Stimulus-responsive nanopreparations for tumor targeting. Integr Biol 2013;
        5(1): 96-107. [eng.].
        [http://dx.doi.org/10.1039/c2ib20135f] [PMID: 22869005]

[132]   Goldenbogen B, Brodersen N, Gramatica A, *et al.* Reduction-sensitive liposomes from a
        multifunctional lipid conjugate and natural phospholipids: reduction and release kinetics and cellular
        uptake. Langmuir 2011; 27(17): 10820-9. [eng.].
        [http://dx.doi.org/10.1021/la201160y] [PMID: 21819046]

[133]   Safarzadeh E, Sandoghchian Shotorbani S, Baradaran B. Herbal medicine as inducers of apoptosis in
        cancer treatment. Adv Pharm Bull 2014; 4 (Suppl. 1): 421-7.
        [PMID: 25364657]

[134]   Friedman JR, Perry HE, Brown KC, *et al.* Capsaicin synergizes with camptothecin to induce increased
        apoptosis in human small cell lung cancers *via* the calpain pathway. Biochem Pharmacol 2017; 129:
        54-66.
        [http://dx.doi.org/10.1016/j.bcp.2017.01.004] [PMID: 28104436]

[135]   Li H, Krstin S, Wang S, Wink M. Capsaicin and Piperine Can Overcome Multidrug Resistance in
        Cancer Cells to Doxorubicin. Molecules 2018; 23(3): 557.
        [http://dx.doi.org/10.3390/molecules23030557] [PMID: 29498663]

[136]   Mahmud M, Piwoni A, Filipczak N, Janicka M, Gubernator J. Long-circulating curcumin-loaded
        liposome formulations with high incorporation efficiency, stability and anticancer activity towards
        pancreatic adenocarcinoma cell lines *in vitro*. PLoS One 2016; 11(12): e0167787.
        [http://dx.doi.org/10.1371/journal.pone.0167787] [PMID: 27936114]

[137]   Arya G, Das M, Sahoo SK. Evaluation of curcumin loaded chitosan/PEG blended PLGA nanoparticles
        for effective treatment of pancreatic cancer. Biomed Pharmacother 2018; 102: 555-66.
        [http://dx.doi.org/10.1016/j.biopha.2018.03.101] [PMID: 29597089]

[138]   Yan Z, Wang Q, Liu X, Peng J, Li Q, Wu M, *et al.* Cationic nanomicelles derived from Pluronic F127
        as delivery vehicles of Chinese herbal medicine active components of ursolic acid for colorectal cancer
        treatment. RSC Advances 2018; 8(29): 15906-14.
        [http://dx.doi.org/10.1039/C8RA01071D]

[139]   Sharma N, Kumar A, Sharma PR, *et al.* A new clerodane furano diterpene glycoside from Tinospora
        cordifolia triggers autophagy and apoptosis in HCT-116 colon cancer cells. J Ethnopharmacol 2018;
        211: 295-310.
        [http://dx.doi.org/10.1016/j.jep.2017.09.034] [PMID: 28962889]

[140]   El-Far SW, Helmy MW, Khattab SN, Bekhit AA, Hussein AA, Elzoghby AO. Folate conjugated vs
        PEGylated phytosomal casein nanocarriers for codelivery of fungal- and herbal-derived anticancer
        drugs. Nanomedicine (Lond) 2018; 13(12): 1463-80.
        [http://dx.doi.org/10.2217/nnm-2018-0006] [PMID: 29957120]

[141]   Yu D, Ruan P, Meng Z, Zhou J. The Structure-Dependent Electric Release and Enhanced Oxidation of
        Drug in Graphene Oxide-Based Nanocarrier Loaded with Anticancer Herbal Drug Berberine. J Pharm
        Sci 2015; 104(8): 2489-500.
        [http://dx.doi.org/10.1002/jps.24491] [PMID: 26052932]

[142]   Zhang J, Wang Y, Jiang Y, *et al.* Enhanced cytotoxic and apoptotic potential in hepatic carcinoma
        cells of chitosan nanoparticles loaded with ginsenoside compound K. Carbohydr Polym 2018; 198:
        537-45.
        [http://dx.doi.org/10.1016/j.carbpol.2018.06.121] [PMID: 30093032]

[143]   Le PN, Pham DC, Nguyen DH, Tran NQ, Dimitrov V, Ivanov P, *et al.* Poly (N-isopropylacrylamide-
        -functionalized dendrimer as a thermosensitive nanoplatform for delivering Malloapelta B against
        HepG2 cancer cell proliferation. Advances in Natural Sciences: Nanoscience and Nanotechnology
        2017; 8(2): 025014.

[http://dx.doi.org/10.1088/2043-6254/aa5e32]

[144] Elgohary MM, Helmy MW, Abdelfattah EA, *et al.* Targeting sialic acid residues on lung cancer cells by inhalable boronic acid-decorated albumin nanocomposites for combined chemo/herbal therapy. J Control Release 2018; 285: 230-43.
[http://dx.doi.org/10.1016/j.jconrel.2018.07.014] [PMID: 30009892]

[145] Kabary DM, Helmy MW, Elkhodairy KA, Fang J-Y, Elzoghby AO. Hyaluronate/lactoferrin layer-b--layer-coated lipid nanocarriers for targeted co-delivery of rapamycin and berberine to lung carcinoma. Colloids Surf B Biointerfaces 2018; 169: 183-94.
[http://dx.doi.org/10.1016/j.colsurfb.2018.05.008] [PMID: 29775813]

[146] Freag MS, Elnaggar YS, Abdelmonsif DA, Abdallah OY. Stealth, biocompatible monoolein-based lyotropic liquid crystalline nanoparticles for enhanced aloe-emodin delivery to breast cancer cells: *in vitro* and *in vivo* studies. Int J Nanomedicine 2016; 11: 4799-818.
[http://dx.doi.org/10.2147/IJN.S111736] [PMID: 27703348]

[147] Barani M, Mirzaei M, Torkzadeh-Mahani M, Nematollahi MH. Lawsone-loaded Niosome and its antitumor activity in MCF-7 breast Cancer cell line: a Nano-herbal treatment for Cancer. Daru 2018; 26(1): 11-7.
[http://dx.doi.org/10.1007/s40199-018-0207-3] [PMID: 30159762]

[148] Singh N, Sachdev A, Gopinath P. Polysaccharide functionalized single walled carbon nanotubes as nanocarriers for delivery of curcumin in lung cancer cells. J Nanosci Nanotechnol 2018; 18(3): 1534-41.
[http://dx.doi.org/10.1166/jnn.2018.14222] [PMID: 29448627]

SUBJECT INDEX

A

Aberrant 7, 73
  activity 7
  EGFR expression 73
Ability 36, 48, 49, 53, 55, 58, 60, 68, 72, 88,
    91, 116, 117, 118, 119, 126
  distinct 117
  enhanced 53
  inducing 126
Absorption 86, 87, 88, 92, 95, 109, 123
  complete 123
  systemic 86, 87
Absorptive cells, intestinal 87
Accelerated cell apoptosis 51
Acid 42, 44, 48, 49, 51, 53, 106, 109, 110,
    111, 114, 122, 125, 126
  acrylic 122
  carbonic 106, 122
  gambogic 48, 51, 53
  hyaluronic 44, 109, 110, 126
  -labile carbamate linkage 114
    linoleic 49
  nucleic 42, 111, 114
  polyarabic 109
  -targeted liposomes 111
  ursolic 125
Actin rearrangement 7
Activated pathway, aberrant 2
Activating JAK mutations 4
Activation 2, 3, 6, 7, 8, 9, 13, 14, 18, 70, 73,
    74, 125, 126
  abnormal 2
  caspase 126
  consequent 6
  constitutive 2
  feedback 13
  increased downstream 6
Active 42, 72
  immunotherapy targets 72
  targeting of nanomedicine 42
Activity 5, 6, 7, 13, 14, 17, 18, 20, 40, 55,
    111, 112, 119, 125
  anti-metastatic 40

cytostatic 13
demonstrated high antiproliferation 55
displayed decreased PTEN 7
minor immunosuppressive 13
Agents 38, 41, 42, 67, 73, 74, 77, 78, 84, 86,
    107, 109, 113, 115, 116, 117, 120, 123,
    124, 125, 127
  anti-angiogenic 73, 113
  commercial gadolinium-based contrasting
    109
  herbal 116, 125, 127
  natural 127
  novel 41
  reducing 123
  surface-active 86
  therapeutic 42, 77, 107, 115, 123
Air pollution 68
Akt downstream targets 11
Akt inhibition 10, 11, 12, 19, 20
  targeted 12
ALK 69, 73
  gene 69
    mutations 73
    -positive metastatic NSCLC 69
Alternating magnetic field (AMF) 116
American cancer society 37
Amino terminal fragment (ATF) 110
Anaplastic lymphoma kinase (ALK) 69, 74,
    77
Androgen receptor (ARs) 117
Angiogenesis 41, 52, 70, 73, 105
  complex 105
Angiogenesis process 106
Animal oils 88
Anti-angiogenic activity 52
Anti-angiogenic effect 73
Antibody 118, 119, 120
  based system 118
  -dependent cellular cytotoxicity (ADCC)
    119, 120
  drug conjugates (ADCs) 120
Anticancer activity 40, 49, 114, 126
  effective 49
  multimodal 40

Anticancer drugs 58, 86, 87, 91, 93, 122, 123,
    127
  lipophilic 91
Anti-cancer Therapeutics 45, 46, 47, 50, 51,
    53, 54, 56, 57, 58, 88
  lipophilic 88
Anticancer therapy 85
Anti-EGF antibodies 2
Antigens 72, 68, 78, 119
  associated 72
  carcinoembryonic 68
  targets TRAIL R1 119
Anti-HER2 antibody 123
Anti-leukemic 11
  action 11
Antisense 57, 59, 76
  oligodeoxynucleotides 57
  oligonucleotides results 76
  technology 59
Anti-synergistic effect 14
Anti-transferrin receptor 112
Antitumor 44, 45, 48, 91, 116, 122, 125
  antibodies 116
  effects 44, 45, 48, 122
  efficacy 44
  properties 91
  treatment efficiency 125
Antitumor activity 48, 52, 56, 116, 127
  improved 52
  increased 56
Antitumoral action 13
Apoptosis 5, 6, 7, 8, 9, 10, 11, 13, 14, 43, 44,
    45, 49, 53, 54, 55, 58, 75, 76, 116, 125,
    126
  accentuated 14
  activity 116
  caspase-dependent 10
  caspase-independent 14
  cellular 11
  higher 49, 53, 54
  increased 54
  induced 116
  inducing 9
  inhibitor survivin 59
  reduced 58
Aptamers 39, 42, 56, 111, 117, 118
  advanced DNA 118
Arematrix-based systems 43
Asthma 73, 126
ATP 56, 68

aptamers 56
ATP binding 9, 124
  -binding sites of mTORC1 and mTORC2 9
  cassette 124
ATP binding site 69
  of EGFR 69
ATP-competitive 11, 12
  dual PI3K/mTOR drugs 12
  inhibitor 11
Autophagy 1, 7, 9, 10, 11, 13, 14, 18, 126
  induced 9
  process 7

B

B-cell 3, 4, 14, 120
  mature 3
  leukemias 120
  lymphomas 120
  precursors 3
  proliferation 4
  receptor (BCR) 14
Bifunctional conjugation of nanoparticles 43
Binding 47, 70, 71, 72, 74, 84
  erratic protein 84
  known intracellular 47
Biomarkers 5, 68, 75, 117
  new genetic 5
  putative cancer 75
Biotin receptor 42
Blocks, immune checkpoint inhibitors 72
Blood vessels 41, 42, 106
  formed 41
  healthy 41, 42
Boronic acid 126
BRCA1 expression 46
Breast cancer 36, 37, 38, 39, 41, 43, 44, 45,
    46, 48, 49, 50, 53, 54, 55, 56, 58, 59
  basal-like 38, 39
  cure 36
  invasive 38
  metastasis 55
    metastatic 37, 48
  resistant 49, 54, 56
  therapy 39, 44, 46, 49, 56
    treatment of 36, 37, 38, 39, 41, 43, 45, 50,
      53, 56, 58, 59
Breast cancer cells 38, 44, 47, 48, 53, 55, 56,
    109
  human 56

metastatic 48, 55
non-metastatic 48
positive 55
undetected 38

C

Camptothecin analogues 124
Cancer 1, 2, 12, 13, 14, 20, 36, 37, 38, 48, 53,
    58, 67, 76, 77, 84, 90, 105, 106, 108,
    109, 110, 111, 112, 114, 115, 116, 117,
    118, 119, 120, 121, 125, 126, 127
  chemotherapy 118
  cervical 119
  colon 2, 114, 117, 118, 125, 126
  deaths 36, 84
  endometrial 125
  genes 58, 67
  growth profiles 114
  liver 126
  malignancies 118
  metastatic genitourinary 112
  pancreatic 14, 20, 110, 115
  prostate 110, 117
  resistant 48
  special 37, 38
  therapeutics 76, 90, 121
  therapy 1, 53, 67, 84, 111, 112, 114, 119,
    120, 127
Cancer cell 51, 72, 117, 119
  biology 119
  cytotoxicity 51
  growth 72
  invasion 117
  higher breast 51
Cancer chemotherapeutics 83, 85, 86, 88, 96
  administration of 85, 96
  bioavailable 88
  delivery of 83
Cancerous cells 84, 106, 116
  permitting 84
Capsaicin 124, 125
  herbal alkaloid drugs 124
Carbodiimide reaction 55
Carbon dioxide gas 122
Carcinogenic conditions 120
Carcinomas 2, 37, 38, 74, 120
  acinic cell 38
  basal-like 37
  embryonal 120

  medullary 38
  neuroendocrine 37
  papillary 38
  renal 2
  squamous cell 74
Cardiotoxicity, reduced 58
Cargo, tumor-killing 55
Cascade 15, 55, 71
  generating cell death 55
  signal 71
Cell cycle 5, 8, 14, 43, 49, 75, 76, 126
  arrest 8, 43, 49, 75
  blockade 14
  progression 5
Cell death 2, 8, 11, 13, 14, 16, 57, 72, 76, 126
  dependent 13
  induced 2
  marked 16
  programmed 11, 14
  programmed tumor 72
Cell growth 1, 6, 8, 13, 16, 37, 72, 75
  abolished 16
  control cancer 72
  suppressing tumoral 13
  suppress leukemic 1
  unregulated 37
Cell lines 13, 44, 48, 54, 55, 57, 59, 76, 111,
    117, 124
  human breast cancer 54, 59
  metastatic cancer 57
  negative human breast 55
  positive human breast cancer 55
  prostate cancer 111
Cells 14, 36, 37, 38, 39, 45, 53, 57, 58, 59, 67,
    72, 73, 74, 87, 106, 112, 115, 116, 117,
    118, 124
  bronchi 73
  carcinogenic 118
  endothelial 73, 106, 124
  healthy 36, 45, 53, 72, 106, 112, 115
  immune 106
  inflammatory 106
  intestinal 87
  metastatic 117
  non-malignant 106
  non-targeted 38
  single 37
  tumour 116
Cellular internalization 44, 55
  higher 55

Cellular processes 70, 75
  basic 75
Cellular progression regulator 7
Cellular uptake 43, 44, 46, 49, 50, 51, 52, 55,
    59, 91, 110, 112, 115, 122, 125
  complex showed higher 122
  higher 43, 44, 50, 55
  increased 49, 51
  insufficient 125
Cell uptake 45, 51, 53, 114, 121
  displayed higher 114
  higher 45, 51, 53
  increased 121
Chemo-photothermal therapy 49
  synergized 49
Chemotaxis assays 55
Chemotherapeutics 41, 74, 86
  normal 74
  traditional 41
Chemotherapy 2, 15, 21, 36, 37, 38, 39, 67,
    74, 75, 84, 85, 86, 113, 115, 122, 124,
    127
  conventional 15, 21, 36, 124, 127
  cycles 113
   high-intensity 21
  local 115
  neoadjuvant 38
  oral 85, 86
  platinum-containing 74
   resistance 2
Chimeric antibody 119, 120
Chinese hamster ovary (CHO) 119
Chitosan 44, 46, 51, 56, 111, 121, 126
  glycol 121
  low molecular weight 111
  nanoparticles 46, 126
  -PLGA micelles 51
  systems 44
  thiolated 44
CHO cells 56
Chromatin 5, 74
  remodelling 74
  structure modifiers 5
Chromosomal 2, 4
  lesions 4
  rearrangement 2
Chronic lymphocytic leukemia (CLL) 9, 18,
    119, 120
Chronic myeloid leukemia (CML) 2, 15
Chrysin's effects 44

Cigarette consumption 68
Circulating tumor cells (CTCs) 118
Circulation 48, 87, 121
  entero-hepatic 87
  plasma 48
Cisplatin 73, 74, 86, 91, 92
  free 92
  minimized 91
Cleavable bond 123
Clonogenic assay 116
Coating, polyarabic acid 109
Colloidal systems 47
Colon cancer cells 2
Colorectal cancer 122, 125
  metastatic 122
Combination 3, 8, 9, 15, 16, 18, 20, 21, 38, 72,
    73, 77, 112, 113, 122, 124, 125
  pharmacological 3
  synergistic 77, 124
Combinational therapy 49
Combination therapy 40, 78
Complement dependent cytotoxicity (CDC)
    119, 120
Complexes 6, 7, 59
  associated signaling 6
  loaded chitosan β-cyclodextrin 59
Concentration-dependent growth inhibition 54
Conjugate 52, 57, 87, 111, 113, 120, 123
  dendrimer LFC131 57
  lipid 111
  lipid-drug 87
  lipid-PEG 52
  nanoparticle-drug 113
  recombinant 120
Conserved family kinases 6
Contemporary research and application 90
Conventional 14, 38, 106
  chemotherapy regimens 14
  dosage forms of chemotherapeutic agents
    38
  drug delivery system 106
Corn oil 90
Cortical-medullary junction 18
CpG-oligodeoxynucleotides function 55
Cremophore 90, 92, 93
  RH40 90, 92
Crk protein 75
Curcumin 48, 49, 50, 51, 91, 92, 93, 116, 125,
    127
  delivery 48, 125

liposomes 125
Cytogenetic profiles 3
Cytokine 16, 23, 58, 116
  encoding immune-stimulatory 116
  genes 116
    inhibitory 58
    receptor 16, 23
Cytoplasmic blebbing 125
Cytosine arabinoside cytarabine 11
Cytotoxic 9, 50, 72, 84, 85, 86, 87, 88, 90, 92, 109, 110
  agents 84, 85, 86
  drugs 87, 88, 90, 92, 109
    oral 85
  effects 9, 50
  peptide 110
  T-lymphocyte 72
Cytotoxic activity 11, 91, 92
  significant 11
Cytotoxicity 45, 49, 91, 119
  antibody-dependent cellular 119
  increased cell 91
  indicated 49
    effect 45

D

Daunorubicin-induced apoptosis 8
Degradation 4, 6, 42, 58, 59, 114
  carbamate link 114
  mediated 4
  nuclease 58
  proteasomic 6
Dendrimer conjugate 54, 55
Dendrimers 39, 40, 43, 54, 55, 56, 57, 58, 76, 106, 107
  aptamers-based 57
  branched oligoethylene glycol 56
  conjugated 55
  developed 54
  grafted polyamidoamide 55
  targeted 55
  targeting 56
  thermoresponsive 54, 56
Diagnosis 39, 76, 84, 105, 106, 107, 108, 109, 111, 118, 124, 127
  antibody-based 118
  early 127
  effective 109
  efficient 111

technology 107
Diagnostic 1, 107
  agent 107
  tools 1
Disease 3, 5, 9, 21, 37, 38, 68, 72, 73, 84, 105, 107, 108, 121, 124, 126
  chronic obstructive pulmonary 73
  complex 37, 38, 107
  deadly 84
  dermatological 126
  heterogeneous 37
  human 5, 68
  minimal residual 3, 21
  multi-factorial 105
  rare 68
DNA 10, 68, 74, 75, 114, 117, 118
  damage, genetic 68
  methylation 74, 75
  methyltransferase inhibitors (DNMTi) 74
  nanoparticles 114
  oligonucleotides 117, 118
  synthesis 10
DNAzyme 58, 59
  delivery 58
  developed mRNA-cleaving 59
DNMT inhibitors 78
Dose-limiting toxicity (DLT) 20, 23, 112, 113
Downregulation 18, 46, 56, 59
DOX 46, 55, 56, 121, 122
  and antisense oligonucleotide 46
  controlled delivery of 56, 121
  generation 55
  release of 121, 122
Doxorubicin 9, 10, 19, 43, 59, 86, 87, 109, 110, 114, 116, 123, 125
  delivery of 109, 116
  loaded 114
  pH-responsive 114
  -resistant breast cancer cell line 59
  sensitive 123
Drug delivery 40, 42, 43, 47, 52, 84, 106, 120, 123, 127
  based stimuli-responsive 120
  molecular targeted 84
Drug delivery systems (DDS) 83, 90, 107, 109, 113, 120, 121, 122, 123, 124, 126, 127
  dependent 83, 90
  novel 109, 113
  responsive 107, 121

sensitive 107, 120, 121
Drug-loaded 56, 87
   dendrimer conjugates 56
   nanoparticulate system 87
   nano-particulate system 87
Drug release 43, 52, 95, 121, 122
   effective 121
   influence 95
   kinetics 52
   mediated 122
   triggered 121
Drug-resistance, bypassing 15
Drug response duration 19
Drugs 8, 9, 11, 13, 15, 36, 39, 40, 42, 43, 45,
      48, 49, 52, 53, 60, 67, 69, 73, 74, 77, 75,
      85, 87, 88, 93, 107, 109, 111, 112, 113,
      122, 123, 127
   allosteric 11
   anti-angiogenic 113
   anti-cancerous 123
   anti-VEGF 73
   approved 67, 69, 77
   chemical 67
   chemotherapeutic 8, 36, 39, 52, 60
   encapsulated 78, 123
   entrapped 112
   hydrophobic 39, 45, 88, 109, 111
   immunotherapy 67
   irreversible 93
   oral 69, 88
   signaling pathway 15
   standard chemotherapeutic 11
   synthetic 73
Duocarmycin analogs 120
Dynamic lipolysis 92

E

Early detection 37, 118
   of breast cancer 37
   of Cancer 118
Effective 58, 115
   delivery system 58
   treatment strategy 115
Efficacy 6, 16, 20, 22, 41, 83, 87, 88, 91, 96
   improved drug 87
   increased Dasatinib 16
   oral 83, 88, 91, 96
   reduced 41
   significant 20, 22

EGFR 44, 46, 67, 69, 70, 71, 74
   effects 44
   exon 69
   expression 46
   gene expression 44
   inhibiting human 71
   mutant 69
   mutations in 71, 74
   targeting 70
   tyrosine kinase inhibitors 67
EGFR inhibitors 2, 71
   active 71
   and anti-EGF antibodies 2
Endocytosis 45, 58, 53, 56, 107
   caveolae-mediated 56
   mediated 45, 58
   receptor-mediated 44, 45
Enzymes 57, 86, 87, 120
   common metabolizing 87
   digestive 87
   major phase-II metabolizing 87
   metabolic 87
   overexpressed proteolytic 120
   restriction 57
Epidermal growth factor receptor (EGFR) 2,
      42, 67, 68, 69, 70, 71, 73, 74, 77
Epigenetic changes in lung cancer 67
Epithelial cells 18, 37
   lining 37
Epithelial mesenchymal transition 67
Estrogen 38
   production 38
   receptor 38
Estrogens 37, 38
Etoposide-phospholipid complex (EPC) 91,
      93
Expression 4, 6, 7, 15, 38, 39, 58, 59, 74, 75,
      76, 78
   aberrant 7, 77
   demonstrated suppressed 58
   hMLH1 protein 76
   inhibiting survivin 59

F

Factors 4, 6, 16, 71, 72, 73, 75, 113
   c-mesenchymal-epithelial transition 71
   growth-regulatory transcription 6
   hepatic leukemia 4
   hypoxia-inducible 73

key transcription 75
platelet-derived growth 16
vascular endothelial growth 72, 113
Fibroblasts 106
    associated 106
Fluorescent dye 110, 114, 117
    infrared 110
Fluorescent substrates 125
Focal adhesion kinase (FAK) 14, 16
Folate 39, 42, 110, 111, 115, 126
    -conjugated PEG-solid fat nanoemulsion
        115
    -conjugated phospholipid 111
    receptor 42
Folic acid 43, 47, 48, 53, 110, 111
    coupling 47
    polymer-core lipid-shell 53
Follicular lymphoma (FL) 119
Food and drug administration (FDA) 67, 69,
    70, 71, 72, 73, 74, 77, 116, 118, 119,
    120
Formation, *in-situ* nanoemulsion 90
FOXO transcription factors 6
FTO gene expression levels 46
Fucosylated oligosaccharides 119
Functional DNAs 114, 121
    nucleic acids 114
    polyelectrolyte 121
Functions 6, 7, 18, 39, 48, 56, 58, 59, 68, 76,
    87, 114, 118
    biological 59
    cellular normal 68
    lysosomal 7
    mitochondrial 56
    nuclear 6
    oncogenic 76
    preserving normal immune 18
Fusion method 95, 112
    liposome 112

G

Gene expressions 56, 59, 75, 106
    controlled 75
    regulating 56
Gene polymorphism 68
Gene regulators 67
Genetic 2, 4, 16, 67
    alterations 2
    damage 67

material 4
    rearrangements 16
GI membrane 86
GI-related untoward effect 95
Glioblastoma 14, 20
    multiforme 14
Glycol chitosan (GC) 3, 11, 13, 17, 18, 121
Graphene nanohybrid (GN) 121
Graphene oxide 115, 121
    modified super-paramagnetic 115
    pH-sensitive nanoscale 121
Graphene quantum dot (GQDs) 109

H

Haematological malignancy 22
HeLa cells 54, 115
Hematologic 1, 5, 8, 11
    malignancies 5, 8
    neoplasms 1, 11
Hematopoietic stem cell transplantation
    (HSCT) 15
Hepatocellular carcinoma 2, 14, 20, 117, 122
HepG2 cells 114
    in comparison 114
HER-2 39, 55, 120
    targeting 55
    cell surface protein 120
    receptors 39
Herbal 124
    drugs development 124
    medicines 124
Heterogeneity 77
Heterolipids 83, 88
High 45, 52, 57
    antiproliferation in HER2-positive cells 57
    antitumor activity 52
    cell internalization and strong anti-cancer
        effects 45
Human 42, 45, 92
    cancer cells 92
    epidermal growth factor receptor 42
    serum albumin 45
Hybrid lipid nanoparticles 53, 54
Hydrogel 49, 115
    micelle-based 49
    pH-sensitive 49
    salt-based 115
Hydrogenated 90
    soybean oil flakes 90

vegetable oils 90
Hyperglycemia 11
Hyperthermia 122
Hypoxia 105, 106, 107, 113
    cells, raised 113
Hypoxic areas of tumor cells 106

I

Ideal theranostic systems 107
Imatinib mesylate effect 15
Immature lymphoid cells 1
Immune 37, 59, 72, 74, 116, 119
    action 119
    -stimulatory effects 59
    system 37, 72, 74, 116
    system attack 72
Immunotherapy 67, 72, 84, 116
    active 72
    passive 72
Implantable gel systems 115
Inducing caspase-dependent apoptosis 9
Inducing cell death 14
Infrared spectroscopy 113
Infusion 84, 85, 93, 118
    intermittent intravenous 85
Inhibition 4, 5, 6, 13, 15, 17, 18, 50, 52, 57,
    58, 71, 76, 88, 91, 115
    activity 5
      cytokine signaling 13
    effective 50, 57, 91
    higher kinase 71
    of tumor cell growth 115
Inhibitors 2, 3, 8, 9, 10, 13, 14, 15, 16, 19, 20,
    21, 69, 71, 72, 76, 77, 120
    allosteric 12
    antibody-based 72
    histone deacetylase 21
    microtubule 120
    multikinase 2
    targeted 20
    targeted cascade 3
    targeting first-generation 71
Intensity 111, 123
    fluorescence 111
Interaction 77, 106
    ligand receptor 106
    pembrolizumab target PD-1/PDL-1 77
Interleukin 4, 8
    abrogate 8

receptor 4
Intracellular 59, 75
    restoration 59
    signal pathways 75
Intrinsic anti-cancer activity 47
Invasive blood neoplasm 3
Ionic complexation 115
Iron 109, 114
    -dependent artesunate 109
    oxide nanocrystals 114

K

Kinase 11, 14, 16, 69
    activation loop 69
    focal adhesion 14, 16
Kinase domain 67, 69, 71
    tyrosine 67, 69

L

Leukemia hematological disorders 1
Leukemias 2, 7, 8, 9, 15, 22, 119, 120
    acute 7
    acute myelogenous 120
    acute myeloid 8
    chronic lymphocytic 9, 119
    chronic myeloid 2, 15, 22
Leukemic cells 11
Leukemogenesis 2
Lipids 6, 39, 52, 83, 87, 90, 106, 124
    biocompatible 83, 90
    cationic 52
    dual specificity 6
    photosensitive 124
Liposomal 112, 122, 125
    encapsulation 125
    nanocomplex 112
    system, sensitive 122
Liposomes 40, 52, 76, 105, 106, 107, 111,
    112, 123, 124, 127
    developed 112
    entrapped 111, 123
    modified 112
    reduction 123
    targeted 111
Low density lipoprotein (LDL) 113
Lower critical solution temperature (LCST)
    122

Low molecular weight chitosan (LMWC) 111
Lung cancer 67, 68, 69, 72, 73, 74, 75, 76, 77, 84, 115, 118, 124, 126
  cell 124
  diagnosis of 68, 75
  metastatic 74
  non-small cell 67, 68, 69, 115
Lung carcinoma 67
Luteinizing hormone-releasing hormone (LHRH) 44
Lymphatic transport, intestinal 87
Lymphatic transport pathway, intestinal 88
Lymphocytes 4, 18
Lymphogenesis 5
Lymphoid progenitor cells 3
Lymphomas 20, 21, 119, 120
  non-Hodgkin 119
  refractory 20
Lyophilized preparation 111

M

Magnetic 111, 114, 118
  properties 118
  resonance imaging (MRI) 111, 114
Magnetic nanoparticles 55, 109, 113
  coated 109
  dendrimer-coated 55
  surface-engineered 113
Malignant 2, 3, 8
  cells 2
  hematological disorder 3
  thymocytes 8
Mammary carcinoma tumor 50
Management of hepatocellular carcinoma 117, 122
MAPK pathways 5, 75
Maximum tolerated dose (MTD) 21
Maytansinoids 120
MDR 52, 54
  breast cancer 52
  cancer cells 54
Mechanism 7, 14, 15, 67, 69, 70, 72, 73, 126
  aberrant cellular 14
  inducing programmed cell death 15
  inhibitory 67
  metabolic 7
Membrane 67, 111, 123, 124
  epidermal growth factor receptor 67
  extrusion 111

fusion 124
  organization 123
Metalloproteinase 76
Metastatic NSCLC 69, 72, 73, 74, 78
  harbouring 74
  positive 69
Methotrexate 19, 45, 46, 92
  accumulation 123
Micellar systems 47, 48, 49, 54
Minimal residual disease (MRD) 3, 21
MiRNAs 58, 59, 67, 75, 76, 78
  cancer-causing 67
  oncogene 76
  suppressive 59
Modified 52, 111, 118
  emulsification technique 52
  liposomal preparation 111
  SELEX technique 118
Monoclonal antibodies 72, 74, 77, 78, 117, 119
  human 74
Mono-nuclear cells 21
Monotherapy 113
Multidrug 86
  efflux pumps 86
  resistance protein 86
Multi-drug treatment regimens 84
Multifunction delivery systems 107
Multiple myeloma 120
Mutation harboring cells 15
Mutations 4, 5, 15, 16, 37, 67, 69, 70, 71, 74, 77, 112
  activated JAK 4
  activating 4, 70
  genetic 5
  somatic 4
  substitution 69
Myeloid lineages 3

N

Nanoemulsion 83, 84, 105, 110, 114, 115, 127
  ligand-appended 115
  oil-in-water 114
Nanoencapsulated drugs 76
Nanoparticles 39, 40, 43, 45, 47, 52, 53, 59, 108, 110, 113, 114, 121, 126
  conjugated hollow mesoporous CuS 108
  cyclodextrin 45, 47
  decorated polyethylenimine-PLGA 59

developed 59, 114
encapsulated dextran-coated iron oxide 59
hybrid 39, 43, 52, 53
inorganic 40
lipid core 113
liquid crystalline 126
magnetic iron oxide 110
pH-titratable super paramagnetic Fe2O3 121
silver 40
super paramagnetic iron oxide 121
Nanoparticle systems 40, 44, 59, 114
developed 59
exploiting 44
polymeric 44
Nanoparticle technology 36
Nanoscale graphene oxide (NGO) 121
Nanosystems 40, 52, 53, 54, 76, 121
dendrimer-based 54
hybrid 52, 53
inorganic 40
National institutes of health (NIH) 116
Natural killer T-cells 73
Nature 39, 75, 97, 88, 96
anti-tumorigenic 75
biodegradable 39
lipophilic 87, 88
self-emulsifying 96
Necrotic cancer cells 57
Neoplastic diseases 1
Neo-vascularization, inhibiting 13
Network 2, 9, 18
inhibition 9, 18
stimulation 2
Next generation sequencing (NGS) 4
Nicotine-derived nitrosamine ketone 68
Nilotinib 9, 15, 17
-resistant cells 15
Niosomes 106, 126
NIRF imaging 114
of nanoemulsion 114
Non-Hodgkin lymphoma (NHL) 119
Non-Hodgkin's B-cell Lymphoma 119
Non-small-cell lung cancer (NSCLC) 13, 67,
    68, 69, 71, 72, 73, 74, 76, 77
Non-targeted liposomal preparation 111
Non-targeted liposomes 111
NSCLC 68, 69, 70, 72, 73, 77, 78
advanced EGFR-mutant 70
lung cancer 68

metastatic EGFR T790M mutation
    harboring 69
nonsquamous 72
squamous 73
treatment of 70, 73, 77, 78
Nucleases enzyme 118
Nucleolin, inhibited 118

O

Oleic acid 90
Oligoethylene glycol derivatives 54
Oncogenes 6, 76
Oncogenesis 2, 6
    mechanism 2
Oncogenic MicroRNA in Lung Cancer 75
Ovarian cancer 109, 110, 113, 118
    metastatic 113
Overexpressed cell surface receptors 43
Overexpressing cancer cells 52
Oxygen consumption 106

P

Pancreatic adenocarcinoma (PA) 125
Panobinostat 21
Passive targeting of nanomedicine 41
Pathogenesis 113
Pathway 7, 22, 40, 58, 67, 116, 124
    calpain 124
    cellular 58
    endocytotic 40
    glycolytic 7
    intracellular 22
    oncogenic 116
    signalling 58, 67
PEGylated 53, 124
    liposomes, prepared 124
    octadecyl-quaternized lysine 53
Penetration 76, 91, 92, 109
    enhanced 76
    improved drug 92
Peptides 39, 42, 47, 48, 68, 110, 116, 124
    homing 48
    novel taxane-binding 47
    pro-gastrin-releasing 68
    self-assembling 116
Perifosine 11, 12
    alkylphospholipid 11

Permeability 41, 54, 86, 106, 125
  enhanced 41, 106, 125
  high membrane 54
  limited 86
Permeation 43, 51, 96
  enhanced 43
  improved 51
Pharmacokinetic results 50
Phosphoinositide 5, 6
  -dependent protein kinase-1 6
Phosphorylation 6, 18, 21, 69, 70, 71
  mediated 6
  tyrosine 71
Piper nigrum 124
Platelet derived growth factor receptor beta
    (PDGFRB) 4, 16
PLGA-PEG 43, 44, 45, 46
  bifunctional nanoparticles 45
  copolymer nanoparticles 46
  nanoparticles 44, 46
Polymer-lipid hybrid system 53, 54
Polymers 39, 40, 43, 48, 49, 52, 95, 106, 107,
    113, 114, 121, 122, 125
  conjugated 49
  hydrophilic 107
  synthesized mPEG-PLGA 48
  synthetic 106
Polymorphisms 5
Polyoxyethylene 95
Polyunsaturated fatty acids, exploiting 92
Post-translation repression 59
Precursor 4, 14
  childhood B-cell 4
  -B-cell receptor 14
Pre-systemic metabolism 86
Proapoptotic role 8
Process 60, 88
  material excretion 60
  self-emulsification 88
Progesterone receptor 38
Prognosis 3, 75
Programmed cell death 73
  ligand 73
  protein 73
Protein kinase 6, 68
Proteins 6, 7, 13, 14, 15, 16, 18, 21, 72, 83,
    86, 111, 116
  adaptor 7
  anti-apoptotic MDM2 15
  cleaved caspase-3 apoptotic 16

cytoplasmic transport 86
immunophilin FK506 binding 13
multidrug efflux 83, 86
proapoptotic 18
proapoptotic BIM 14
ribosomal 21
PTEN 6, 8
  and loss of activity 6
  post-translational inactivation 8
PTX nanoemulsion (PNs) 115
Pulmonary hypertension 73
Puma's expression modulation 21

R

Radioisotope, immune 119
RAS protein 75
Reactive oxygen species (ROS) 109, 125
Receptor-mediated endocytosis process 114
Receptor tyrosine kinases 2, 6
Recognition 106, 111, 116
  antibody-antigen 106
Relapsed multiple myeloma 21
Resistance 11, 68, 123
  mutations 68
    oxidative stress 123
  steroid 11
Reticuloendothelial system 42
Rheumatoid arthritis 126
RNA 58, 59, 76, 127
  gene 1-small interference 59
    induced silencing complex (RISC) 76
    interference (RNAi) 58
    therapeutics 127
Rolling circle amplification (RCA) 114
ROS 77, 126
  production 126
  proteins 77

S

Selective estrogen receptor modulator 38
Self 83, 87, 88, 47, 90,9 1, 94
  -assembled chitosan nanoparticles 47
  -emulsification performance 94
  -emulsifying drug delivery system 90, 91
  -nanoemulsifying drug delivery system 83,
    87, 88
Serum urea 92

Signaling 3, 15
   pathway downstream 15
   tyrosine kinases 3
Signal 1, 93, 112
   transduction 1
   -chain antibody fragment 112
   -dose studies 93
   walled carbon nanotubes 127
SiRNA 58, 77
   developed A2AR-specific 58
   nanoencapsualted 77
SiRNA molecules 58
Small 1, 3, 12, 15, 22, 67, 68, 77, 124
   cell lung cancers (SCLC) 67, 68, 77, 124
   molecule inhibitors (SMIs) 1, 3, 12, 15, 22
   -molecule kinase inhibitors 68
Solidification 94, 95
   process 95
   techniques 94, 95
Solid tumors 1, 14, 20, 112, 120
Src family kinases 7
Stimuli 6, 105, 106, 107, 114, 115, 120, 121, 122, 123, 127
   endogenous 127
   external magnetic 123
   extracellular 6
   magnetic 123
    sensitive drug delivery systems 120
    -triggered drug delivery systems 127
Suppress feedback activation 15
Surfactants 83, 87, 88, 90, 93, 95
   toxic 93
Synergetic effect 49
Synergism 10, 14, 16, 17
Synergistic action 112
Synthetic macromolecular structures 54

T

Target 48, 58
   breast cancer 48
   cancer cells 58
Targeted therapies 1, 2, 68
   developing new 2
   molecular 68
Targeting breast cancer 115
Taxane-binding peptide (TBP) 47
T-cell progenitors 5, 18
   immature 5
T-cells 3, 72, 73, 120

lymphoblastic 3
Temperature sensitive drug delivery systems 122
Theranostic 107, 114, 118
   system 107, 114
   monoclonal antibodies 118
Therapies 12, 37, 38, 44, 48, 49, 58, 68, 74, 78, 84, 85, 105, 109, 114, 116, 127
   cytotoxic 84
   directed 114
   effective 44
   epigenetic 74, 78
   first oncolytic virus 116
   gene transfer 116
   hormonal 38, 84
   immunosuppressant 105
   implementing gene 58
   photodynamic 109
   photothermal 49, 109
Transferases 87
Transferrin receptor 42
Transformation 3,4, 7
   impaired leukemic 7
   leukemia cells 4
Translocations 4
   reciprocal 4
   variant 4
Trastuzumab 39, 55, 57, 72, 120
   emtansine 120
   synthesized 55
Treatment 60, 77, 84, 108, 115, 125
   combinatorial 108
   conventional breast cancer 60
   effective 125
   effective cancer 84
   localized cancer 115
   single drug 77
Triple negative breast cancer (TNBC) 39, 43
Tuberous sclerosis 7
Tumor cells 40, 42, 52, 72, 73, 74, 106, 107, 109, 112, 114, 116, 118, 124, 125
   circulating 118
   proliferation 52, 109
   targeted malignant 124
Tumor growth 13, 38, 49, 50, 56, 59, 70, 73, 74, 105, 109, 115, 122
   -inhibition effect 50
   inhibiting 49
   reduced 50
   support 70

suppressed 115
Tumors 37, 38, 39, 40, 41, 42, 44, 47, 48, 52,
      53, 54, 57, 68, 77, 106, 109, 117, 122,
      124
   breast 54, 57
   gastrointestinal 117
   induced 44
   initial 37
   ncerous 68
   overexpressed 52
Tumor suppressor gene 2, 6, 76, 74, 75, 112
   inhibiting 76
      phosphatase 2
      upstream 6
Tumor suppressor(s) 75, 76
   MicroRNAs in Lung Cancer 75
Tumor vasculature 55, 106
   restricted 106
Tumor vasculature cells 106
Turbid emulsions 94
Tyrosine kinase 1, 3, 9, 15, 16, 67, 68, 69, 70
   activity 68, 69
   inhibitors (TKIs) 1, 3, 9, 15, 16, 67, 70
TZ-conjugation of dendrimers 55

U

Ubiquitin ligase 6
Upper critical solution temperature (UCST)
      122
Uptake 47, 107, 113
   intracellular 47
   macrophagic 113
   reticulo-endothelial system 107
Ursolic acid (UA) 125

V

Vascular endothelial growth factor (VEGF)
      72, 73, 75, 113
   receptor (VEGFR) 73
VEGF 2, 55, 111
   -antisense oligodeoxynucleotides 55
   gene expression 111
   /RAF/RAS pathway 2
Venous catheter 85
Vessels, lymphatic 52
Viability 9, 18, 96
   cellular 9

preserving lymphocyte 18
Vincristine 9, 11, 16, 20, 43, 45, 86
   sulfate 43, 45
Viruses 116, 117
   non-oncolytic 116

W

Weighted magnetic resonance contrast agent
      121
Western blot 116, 126
   study 126
   technique 116

X

Xenobiotics 87, 88